Jenny Eats the World

Tales of a Traveling Bulimic

By

Jennifer Martin

CONTENTS

DEDICATION

To my grandmother, Joanne. You have been my biggest cheerleader in my writing, encouraging me to pursue this career since the dawn of my first blog. Thank you for always believing in my abilities, and for raising three loving, caring, intelligent children.

ACKNOWLEDGMENTS

To my father, Frank Martin, who has been sober all my life. Thank you for staying committed to your health, your career and in doing so, your family. Thank you for providing me with an education and the editor who helped me refine this book. You are the only person who I am afraid of reading this memoir, as I share stories no father would want to read about their children. Please have grace.
I love you.

To my mother, Laurie Martin. Who raised my brother and I with love, grace, and a can-do attitude. Thank you for always putting healthy food on our table, for taking us to sports practice, and for taking care of yourself so you could show up for us. You may not have the disease of addiction, but your soul chose to love a family of addicts, and I'm so fortunate for that.

To my editor, Jaimee Garbacik. You were my editor, my therapist and my life coach all wrapped up in one thorough review. Never did I ask myself *why* when I wrote my first draft, and you helped me see far between the lines of my life. Editing the second draft of this book with your notes allowed me to see my biases, my privilege, and myself through my story in a transformative way.

To my coach, Tessa Faye. YOU ROCK. No one has believed in my abilities more than you have. I am honored to know you and lucky to work with you. And I'm excited, knowing this is only the beginning.

DISCLAIMER

The content in this body of work is for entertainment and educational purposes only. I am not a doctor, a dietitian, a psychologist, nor a specialist of any sorts. But I do find my story special enough to share and compose into the book you hold in your hands today.

Please do not substitute my story for the professional advice of a licensed physician or health care provider. If you are inspired to take action after reading this book, more power to you. I cannot take responsibility for the actions of which you take. Whatever you decide to do, please respect yourself and others.

Note that all statements in this book are based on the opinions and observations of Jennifer Martin. For obvious privacy reasons, names and details of the people and institutions mentioned in this book have been changed. Everything about this story is true.

I cannot guarantee any results or changes in your mental, physical, emotional, or spiritual well-being by reading this book. I do, however, truly hope that my story evokes courage within you to lead a more authentic life.

This book contains strong language and adult content that may not be suitable for unsupervised children. Discussing such topics of this book with your children in a safe and educational environment is, however, encouraged when such children reach an appropriate age.

Consider this your trigger warning.

Me, Myself and Ed

If I could have my cake and eat it too, then none of this would have happened. If I could have my cake like a no-strings-attached, one-time-fling, then I would have never developed such a toxic relationship with Ed. If only I could eat cake like a normal person, then the past decade would have likely been more orthodox than the events that I share with you today. However, when I have my cake, I fantasize over my cake. I lust over my cake. I devour my cake until there is no crumb left behind.

For years, cake, or all food for that matter, controlled my life. As if the motor functions for my hands and mouth were programed to grab, chew, and swallow as much food as possible, white knuckling between each vanishing act. Counselors and psychologists would call my relationship with food an eating disorder, but I like to personify this bond as "Ed." Ed was my longtime partner throughout college and my early twenties, although I cheated on him ad nauseum. Even so, those love affairs only brought me closer to Ed, strengthening my dependence on him before relying on a higher power for self-assurance.

Originally, Ed labeled cake as the enemy. He whispered sweet nothings into my ear, urging me to avoid cake at all costs. In college, my weight was at an all-time low while my exertion was at an all-time high. Competing as a Division I swimmer, I scribed the calorie count of every egg white I ate between three-hour practices along the ribs of my notebook. My plate was judged consistently by teammates as they compared my salad to their double servings of something more savory than romaine. As for my male counterparts, their caloric intake left me basking in awe and envy. They achieved their six-pack abs with six-packs of beer and stayed lean despite their religious late-night "fourth meal." Throughout college, my source of carbs largely consisted of alcohol, which helped me reach my daily allotment of 1,800 calories each night with a 400 calorie can of malt liquor. Prior to the FDA's intervention on the original Four Lokos, those candy-colored cans of fermented caffeine nursed me through my first semester.

Prior to university, I was your average good girl. Growing up in the suburbs of Kansas City, I was a high-achieving athlete who made respectable grades. I wasn't drinking (much) and remained a virgin to both drugs and *the deed*. In those first three years of high school my world revolved around swimming. Much had shifted since adolescence, when I begged my parents to drop me off at a cold pool at the crack of dawn, insisting to return after sundown. But the more my hair faded into green, my enthusiasm for the sport dwindled down to a chore as swimming only seemed to be my ticket into college.

Once I reached senior status, my positive perception as an athlete morphed into the fear of being a living, breathing Troll Doll. For years, my distinguishable wet head and embedded goggle marks accessorized my swim meet apparel. Those tee shirts may not have been as fashionable as Abercrombie & Fitch, but my name was printed on my back. Being "cool" was not my top priority as long as I was *special*.

At practice, however, "special" was the name of a set derived from hell. Only the girl who went on to win a medal at the London Olympics was special. Built like a deity from another planet. The rest of us accepted our mortality by making sexual whale noises between sets and tickling the toes of our antecedent lane mates. The pool was an ecosystem I could thrive in, with other masochistic teens with dreams of scholarships and split ends.

When trying to code-switch from the pool to school, I didn't always click with the cliques. While I could talk to anyone, I never felt like I truly *fit in*. Girl groups were merely a teenage fantasy in which I wanted no part in the play. My fantasy was always to swim at Stanford. And while I was

2

good, I was not good enough and Stanford became just another place in California. In accepting this, suppressed ideations of joining a sorority began to surface in response to my deep-seeded desire: *to belong*.

When college applications started rolling out, I decided to take a step back from a sport that now felt obligatory. I teetered between choosing four years of themed parties and social recognition, and the student-athlete lifestyle I was already accustomed to. The allure of rush and the glamorization of Greek life spurred my obsession with monogramming my closet, although my wardrobe consisted of mostly sportswear. Torn, I was unwilling to relinquish eight years of swallowing chlorine just to shot-gun beers in the cement basement of a frat house. I did, however, end up shot-gunning copious beers in dingy basements, just with less trust fund kids wearing Vineyard Vines.

After extensive contemplation regarding the dread of mediocrity, I committed to swimming at a private university in Cincinnati, Ohio, before embarking on my last semester of high school. This commitment was a meager attempt to retaliate burnout. I began to dread the sport, but I was not ready to give up on my childhood dreams. Anticipating practices provoked angst and anxiety, even short-term panic. I loathed practice, yet without it, I would find myself at a loss. So, I compromised. I cut down. My training, my competitions, and inevitably, my eating. With this decision, my relationship to food and exercise entered an entirely new era. A world of which hosted the parasite, Ed. The honeymoon period with Ed began like any cautionary tale of anorexia, in that Ed and I started dating by going on a diet. I saw the scale creeping up senior year, so once my weekly training tapered from 30 to 20 hours in the pool with significantly easier sets, I cut out all junk food. I swapped three-hour swim practices for five-mile runs, in addition to a ninety-minute swim after a dinner free of carbs. I let myself snooze until 7am, as opposed to 4:20. I traded chicken tenders and fries for packed lunches in my ever so trendy Vera Bradley lunch bag and stopped eating a sleeve of Oreos as an after-school snack. From this drastic diet change and extra rest, pounds fell off fast. Looking back, being seventeen and sober was a probable factor in my 'fast' metabolism, whatever that means. Though as I shed weight at a steady rate, I seemed to be the only one to notice. Fast forward to March, when I had four impacted wisdom teeth removed after an all-inclusive spring break in Mexico. And as fast as one sips a yard stick at Señor Frogs, I said "adios" to all that was normal in my life.

What a cliché, right? An innocent teen looking to slim down slips into disease after oral trauma: a convenient excuse not to eat, to stick to a liquid diet, to point blame for rapid weight-loss. Unfortunately for me and fortunately for Ed, my history of oral health has never impressed any dental professional, as I encountered serial dry sockets and infections for weeks after surgery. Going to class became a hassle as freshmen gawked at my chubby cheeks during the passing period. I did not mind the stares, but I couldn't tolerate the pain. By graduation, I totaled up 88 absences in a single year. Unlike the previous years where any leave was due to a swim meet, I called out 88 times to doze off at home when the pain peaked, and the Vicodin kicked in. Correction: my mom called me out 88 times. She's the true MVP.

Mom never swam competitively, unlike my best friend Alyssa. However, like my mom, Alyssa also grew concern for my shrinking physique.

"Jenny!" A chill ran down my neck as Alyssa's eyes burned into my skin. My gangly legs bowed in front of the water fountain, where she confronted me half naked in my Speedo.

"I can see every bone in your back."

I stood up straight to wrap my scapula around those bony bits. Perhaps better posture would soften the harsh edges of my protruding spine. I turned to face my freckled and fair skinned friend, with her golden ringlets draping along her face.

"Yea, so, I lost some weight. I had dry sockets for like a month."

"Jenny. People are noticing. Cara Sinclair asked about you. She said you're "disappearing."

I looked down and smirked in agitation.

"I'm not going anywhere. Except for practice, of which, we're now late."

For someone who was disappearing, I was gaining a considerable amount of attention.

Despite my twenty-five-pound weight loss from an already athletic build, I still didn't consider myself *that* skinny. I was seventeen. Hardly half of my class had boobs. The other half kept complimenting me - *noticing me* - for the first time. The few who truly knew me asked if I was doing ok.

Why would I not be ok? Was it not ok to eat baby carrots for dinner after hours of cardio? Doesn't everyone know the exact number of calories in their lunch box? Who doesn't panic after eating a cookie, then runs through stairwells when taking a bathroom break?

How dare Clara Sinclair claim that I'm disappearing. I'm still here! I could only confide in my internalized friend, Ed, who reassured me these remarks were the finest of compliments.

Ed made sure I avoided red meat, always ordered salad - hold any nuts or cheese and keep the dressing on the side. If I were to have something of the sweet or savory variety, Ed and I sweat out every morsel of my misbehavior. Sometimes running in the dead of night to keep my parents at bay. They never suspected I was sneaking out to drink booze or smoke doobies. No, my surreptitious escapes were far less social but just as dangerous. If for whatever reason I could not find time for a second workout, Ed prescribed me a dose of laxatives. As prom season approached, I flaunted my medicinal remedy to Alyssa like someone might praise their success in any weight-loss program:

"Just pop a Dulcolax a couple of nights before the dance. That's what I'm doing so my zipper doesn't break at dinner again."

"And we have string together safety pins to keep your dress on at The Capital Grille? That was hilarious." Allyssa said innocently.

"O god..." I laughed with Alyssa, only to hear Ed remind me of this humiliating account from my Junior Prom. Though a year ago, I was undaunted by this wardrobe mishap. Those broad shoulders of mine kept breaking personal records - let them break a zipper or two. However, this flashback now inundated my self-esteem with despair. I was desperate to keep shrinking.

After months of tanning beds, liquid diets, excessive exercise and the occasional laxative, prom night finally arrived. My 00 gown wrapped around my 5'7' frame which now carried 119.3 pounds. When a dozen groomed teenagers posed in front of a family room fireplace to capture the years' most liked Facebook photo, my scrawny arm caught more attention than my dress.

"Jenny! You've gotten so skinny!" One mom shouted behind her Canon PowerShot. I would hear that word a dozen more times throughout the night, beaming brighter with every accreditation. But soon following the dance, that "skinny" label transformed, becoming a burden, a negative connotation, and a major concern for my parents.

The next week in government class, an abrupt message blared from the intercom. "Jennifer Martin to the counselor's office." Twenty white faces turned at me, but I brushed them off like I had half of my attendance that semester. I figured the inquiry was related to college enrollment. But as I approached the office, slivers of my mom, dad, and high school swim coach waited for me behind the opaque glass walls. I treaded gingerly.

"Um, hey." I whispered as time and space slowed down around the room. The lingering apprehension among the adults worried me. Has a family member died? Why was my coach there? Finally, my counselor, a woman whom I had little relationship with besides our biannual class registration, broke the silence.

"Jenny," she said calmly with a soft stare from her light blue eyes. I, on the other hand, sat rigid in my seat, squeezing my palms between my bony knees to avoid any fidgeting.

"We brought you in here because we're worried about your weight."

Damn.

Let's dive straight into the action, forget foreplay. I sat in shock, offended by a comment I took as an accusation.

Well, at least nobody died.

"Uh… what do you mean?" I tried to cover my irritation with false ignorance.

"Jenny! Look at you!" cried my mom.

"You're too skinny!"

Ugh, that word again. I wasn't skinny, I was thin. Skinny girls don't play sports. Skinny girls can't sustain three-hour swim practices...

My coach intervened: "Jenny, your weight loss has affected your season dramatically. I don't see the stamina and the power in the pool this year."

He had a point. My times were suffering at meets, despite how I led the lane at practice.

"But I'm not getting dizzy or anything. I'm eating enough. I promise."

The counselor stepped in: "Your classmates have expressed that you're only eating vegetables at lunch and abusing laxatives."

Damnit, Alyssa.

"No, no, I've just been on a health kick since I started packing my lunch. I mean, I was eating fries every day, and now I'm not, so you think I'm anorexic? I don't abuse laxatives, I just get irregular on my period."

My face froze to stone in that last lie, as my period had become dangerously light, and often failed to come at all. I pulled out every excuse to avoid the inevitable: a plea for weight gain.

My dad's fists flatted as he softened in his seat. He sighed and stared at the corner of the room, about to speak up on something he had been battling to express for weeks.

"Your mom and I want you to see a professional to help you regain what you've lost since having your wisdom teeth pulled."

There it was, the threat against Ed: *We just want you to gain weight. Fatten up. Undo all the hard work you've put into earning your lean body.*

By now, I could not differentiate my voice from Ed's, who held my hand throughout the intervention. I didn't want to gain weight, but I didn't want to disappoint my coach or my parents either. I agreed to see a dietician, partially to earn brownie points from the adults, but also to quiz the health professional about her career. Considering how much I studied nutrition labels, I was practically a couple credits in towards earning my RDN. What career could be more appropriate for someone who thought about food 99% of the day?

In fact, that statistic was the first thing she asked me.

"How many times a day do you think about food?" the dietician began. The wall of science books and other texts written by authors with half a dozen initials by their name still did not convince me that this woman could use her wits on my willpower to keep eating as I damn pleased.

What do you mean how many times? I think about food as much as I breathe.

"Um… Just before meals, like when I'm hungry" I lied.

"How much water, coffee, and diet drinks do you consume in a day?"

I lifted my 500mL water bottle, hypothesizing an honest answer.

"Maybe one of these, every other class, plus refills during and after practice, so about 3-4 Liters a day, plus two cups of coffee in the morning, and diet sodas on the weekends."

"That's quite a lot of calorie-free liquid, which is a major appetite suppressant," she said while scribbling in her notebook as we sized one another up. Staring off at all her psychology books, my mind spun around the vast information I had yet to uncover *about* the mind. Reading titles around eating disorders, I scoffed a look of disapproval from my rigid seat on the couch.

"Bitch" I thought.

"Bitch" thought Ed.

I tried laughing off her assumption. "I sweat a lot. Probably more than most people. I can lose up to four pounds of water weight in one swim practice."

"How often do you weigh yourself?" She responded swiftly.

Damnit. She got me.

I couldn't tell her the truth of my persistent weigh-ins. I couldn't tell her how Ed monitored the number every morning. Best case scenario, he'd pat me on the back for a respectable number and allow some wiggle room on the day's calorie count - assuming I would wiggle it off. Other times, I would shiver on the white square in humiliation as Ed assailed the digits in front of my toes, pinching at my stomach, my arms, and my hips. On those days, I would hang my head low on the bathroom scale like a dog whimpering beside a torn pillow, waiting for my master to scold me for taking a bite of something I should not have chewed.

I sat in silence for a moment, gathering an appropriate response to her interrogation.

"I weigh myself on Sundays at my dad's gym when he takes me to a yoga class." My heart raced under an inscrutable face.

"And how much do you exercise?" She asked, despite her knowledge of my swimming background.

This question was easy, considering my answer was well-rehearsed. Swimming and other sports occupied my childhood, and I loved nothing more than to boast about the details of my athletic endeavors. I sat up taller and spoke clearer, rattling off a typical evening after school at the gym, followed by dinner, followed by swim practice. For the average person, my sweat-sessions may seem outlandish and overindulgent. But for an elite swimmer, my training was sub-par. The dietician's main concern seemed to be that my appetite mirrored that of an average person, not an athlete. Our hour ended and the dietician suggested drinking fortified protein shakes between meals. Ed and I left the office in frustration, interpreting our hour-long session as a simple order: "Eat more."

I drove home an optimist, thankful I wouldn't have to lie to my parents about any major concerns or diagnoses the dietician might have and I could tell them confidently that there was no need to worry. But to my surprise, they did not express any worry when I returned home that Saturday afternoon. They acted as if they had forgotten about the appointment *they* scheduled without my consent. As I waited for them to berate me with questions, my optimism morphed into paranoia. Surely, the dietician had already contacted my parents with an in-depth report of our meeting, proclaiming an initiative to fatten me up!

After reeling through a couple worst-case scenarios around my weight gain, my mom broke her attention from Candice Olson on HGTV and asked: "So how was it?"

Back came the optimism.

"It was great! I learned a lot. There's a ton of science involved in becoming a registered dietician, though, so I'm not sure if I want to take that route in college." I said, pointedly avoiding my mom's intended question.

"But what did she say about *you*, Jenny?" Another gray hair grew on her head of faded red. The interrogation shifted into a sigh of irritation.

"Oh. She said I eat very healthy. That I should add in some meal replacement foods as snacks to make sure I'm getting enough protein."

My mom shrugged, "Ok."

I perked up, "Ok!"

Phew. Glad *that* was over. My mom returned to studying DIY projects on HGTV and I went on to study the macronutrients of Boost shakes and Cliff bars.

Despite my efforts to slurp on protein isolates, my swimming performance tanked during my last high school state meet. It was the first competition where I failed to qualify for the finals in an individual race, leaving me to share the spotlight with my relay team on the awards stand. I shivered in tears on that podium, swallowing the bittersweet ending of my high school swimming career. The Kansas state meet fell a day before graduation, and everything I knew which was comfortable and convenient was withering away. To simulate a sense of control, I committed myself to shed every ounce gained from those damn shakes. Leaving high school behind, I would reclaim myself as I entered what I expected to be "the best four years of my life."

The first week of those best-four-years rolled out slowly with a road trip accompanied by my parents, who helped me move into my dorm during orientation. As we toured campus, passing students spoke of hangovers and keg stands as my family and I approached the bookstore, which made my dad's eyes roll and my mother blurt out: "Oh brother..."

Speaking of brothers, it was time to resurface a salient topic my parents once had with me and Matt when we started high school. It was *the talk* I'd imagine most parents dread having, don't have, or regret not having after it's too late. No, I'm not speaking of sex here. Rather, what it means to *drink responsibly.*

During that talk, my parents sat Matt and I down in the living room to discuss why Dad doesn't drink. My dad placed his worn, tan hands in his lap, staring at his feet as my brother and I sat in apprehension on the couch.

"I'm sure you've noticed, but I'm not so sure how much you two are aware." My dad's tone dropped, entering lecture mode.

"I'm an alcoholic. And because I'm an alcoholic, I don't drink."

My brother and I held our breath as our dad stared at us stoically. We were surely *aware* that dad never grabbed beers with the other parents after sporting games, but we never really knew *why*.

"Drinking got me into a lot of trouble when I was your age. As an adult, it really messed up my life. I've been arrested, charged with DUI's, and kicked out of bars from starting fights. This isn't to scare you or to say you'll face the same consequences I had. What I'm saying is that alcoholism is a gene, and you two are predisposed to the gene."

Dad sat his hands back in his lap. His lecture was over. As a woman who stops at one, maybe two drinks per event she occasionally drinks at, my mom shook her head in sympathy, took a deep breath and chimed in:

"Addiction is so ugly, isn't it?"

Standing in an old dorm room that was new to me, my parents crowded around my bunk bed for the final goodbye after reviewing spark notes of *the talk*. My parents never told me what to do, but they warned me of what might happen if I drank like my dad. I didn't listen. Even in the dorm room, where I had already snuck in a bottle of Smirnoff, my parents understood they had to relinquish all control over a college custom that I'd inevitably and enthusiastically engage in. No, my parents didn't need to tell me to be careful with alcohol, they said it all with one sober stare:

"You have the gene, Jen."

I squeezed them both goodbye before ushering them out of the dorms. I promised them I'd be careful. I promised myself that I wouldn't drink like my dad and have to get sober, trading parties for church basements because I can drink like a lady. I wanted to prove to myself and all my new college peers that despite any predispositions, Jennifer Martin could hold her liquor.

With my family's history of addiction in mind, I was cautious of crossing the line between college parting and alcoholic behavior. Which, unequivocally, are the same behaviors. But I was eighteen and had yet to black out or throw up from drinking, thus I perceived my nightly imbibing as a network tactic to make myself known around campus.

After three months of two-a-day practices, I built up an appetite indisputably larger than the fruit-and-salad diet I maintained over the summer. Ed's voice simmered down despite how I was eating bread again, as we both knew my increase of physical exertion allowed for extra calories. I remained the thinnest girl in the pool and was often mistaken for a cross-country runner. Correcting such assumptions always made me smile.

My peers mistook me for a runner as well, as the girlfriends I made outside of the swim team praised my body every night we swapped wardrobes for a house party. I then caught the attention of any guy I wanted at said house parties, elevating my self-esteem higher than my respectable GPA. On campus, I morphed from the skinny swimmer to the social butterfly between the hours of dinner and buzzed o'clock. This balancing act of studies, swim practice and social sprees instilled a feeling of productivity, distracting me from disparaging concerns around food. In my naivety, I was winning at life, as the occasional meatball sub at 1am on a Friday morning had no effect on my weight that I continued to monitor. Ed was now an ex I dumped in high school. I was on my own now. I was golden.

Though left unmaintained, precious metal begins to wear. And without awareness, my chains of control began to rust. My golden shell was simply a facade, and with one single sentence, my veneer exterior vanished into dust.

Upon their arrival in late October, my parents visited campus and studied my physique like I did psychology. While her unintended reversal seemed innocent, my mother's opening line cracked open Pandora's box of anorexic thoughts:

"Wow, Jenny. You look good. Your cheeks are getting fuller!"

Blood rushed into my face that Mom just described as *full*.

I was done for. Scared and exposed, Ed sensed my fear and sent me countless texts, left voicemails, and even wrote on my Facebook wall in hopes of rekindling our relationship. And in my shaken state, I caved.

As Ed demanded more attention, I subconsciously sought out validation from a man more tangible than a conniving voice in my head. No amount of love and support from my parents could suppress Ed. Despite my folks driving across the country to visit me that weekend, every concerning comment kept me in a dark distance.

"You're the smallest one on the team, Jenny." My dad noted at our last dinner together. I stared down at my plate of greens, gripping my fork with white knuckles. Typically, this observation would fuel my self-esteem, but coming from him, I left the restaurant squeamish. He just did not understand. How could he? He's not an eighteen-year-old girl. He's sober, and already killing my buzz. Doesn't he know that I have a party to attend?

I just needed to drink. To forget. To flirt. To finally give in to the guy on the team who keeps flirting with me. And now… now that guy is walking me home, or rather, we are heading back to his. Making out on his couch. Making way to his bed. But we don't do *it*. Because I'm (still) a virgin. I'm waiting for love. And Evan was waiting for me.

This dark-blonde, sleepy-eyed, preacher's kid from Tennessee was a sophomore on the swim team who had wooed me with his wit over the first months of college, leading me into his arms that weekend my parents came to visit. Evan was the first man to plant the seed of a flowering romance, taking his time to water our potential and patient enough to wait and watch us grow. The patience was honorable. The persistence was obligatory, considering we already spent ten hours a week together - wet, sweaty, and nearly naked. Such a cocktail of hormonal influence alchemizes many relationships among teammates and is a phenomenon known as *swimcest*. Reluctant at first to stigmatize my relationship status, I fooled around one final time before I could show up for someone who gave his heart to me.

After four weeks of second (ok, third) base standing with Evan, I had finally caught the attention of the cute, tall, baseball boy who lived in my dorm. My self-esteem was, how you say, *low,* thus my drunken decision to fondle the baseball player on his futon seemed valid despite the stakes being so *high*. Word got around quicker than I did, which, by any standard, is a major foul.

Evan and I were not official, so I convinced myself that I was a free agent. I told myself that if I did not have a "boyfriend," I could kiss whoever I pleased. But what I told myself came out a bit differently when I explained to Evan what happened that night on the futon when we were partying on Halloween:

"I'm just not used to this attention!" I cried into my Solo Cup, after Evan had smashed his down in front of me.

"I don't know… this whole college thing. Partying. Dorm life. It's all so new and overwhelming and I got caught up in the moment because we're not official, but it made me realize that I want to make it official because I care about you…"

I looked up from my Solo Cup to see the back of Evan's head drifting away. Being cute might have caught me a night with the baseball boy but it was not enough to convince Evan to forgive me. (And I was dressed as Buddy the Elf!)

I'd need to apologize and admit my feelings in sobriety. I would need to commit myself to the companionship I so deeply craved. I would need to learn to reciprocate care and appreciation for the first time. And for a stretch of time, I tried.

Young and in love, our conversations surpassed surface level similarities, like our affinity for Tosh.0. Evan encouraged me to find purpose past graduation, to question the norms of what our peers were chasing and emboldened me to view myself as attractive regardless of my appearance. While I had previously dreamed of obtaining my M.R.S. degree in college, dating Evan challenged my hopes of becoming a housewife.

"For someone so beautiful, you don't allow your looks to define you, Jen. That's what sets you apart from the other girls." Evan said one afternoon in late November, just weeks after we decided to see each other exclusively.

I blushed, not knowing how to respond. I recognized my conventional beauty of thick blonde hair and wide hazel eyes. I knew that looks could hold power, but I did not want my appearance to determine my power. I wanted to be pretty *and*. I wanted to be skinny *and*. I wanted attention, but I wasn't exactly sure for what and why. Evan offered his attention. Not to dangle a dainty girl on his arm, but to understand me as someone who now played an important part of his life. Whereas Evan did not strike me as overwhelmingly "hot" at first sight, he had swag. He listened attentively to others and sought to learn more about me. And *that* was sexy.

Evan was the son of a preacher, who was also an attorney. While Evan questioned organized religion after spending his adolescence in church, our earlier spiritual views gelled in that we attended Sunday school to please our parents but did not practice much prayer outside those holy walls. When it came to sex, we had both waited for the right person at the right time. And with every dorm-room date we had after that fretful Halloween night, our passion escalated to a fervor. The concept of deflowering my celibate panties to another virgin whom I trusted and adored was everything I imagined when doing it for "the first time."

The sex itself, however, was ineptly anticlimactic. As in I didn't climax. But we made it so intentional and consensual that my first time was like mist on my skin in a fairy garden opposed to mind-blowing fireworks across a vast field. But thanks to our determined spirit, we spent just as many hours practicing in the bedroom as we did in the pool.

As we neared the end of the swim season that spring, our love for one another swelled from tentative to certainty. But Evan's interest in the sport had ceased, leading him to retire in March after the conference championship. Luckily for us, the remaining two months of the semester served as the swim team's "off-season," a period of reduced hours of training per bylaw of the NCAA. Off-season is something of a Rumspringa for athletes: a chance to engage in common college practices with inconsequential alcohol and drug abuse.

One night after a string of parties, a handful of the men's swim team opted out of booze and instead hit the bong at the "swim house" (a kind of frat house for the swim stars: equally as vulgar and douchey). Evan knew I wanted to "try" getting high since my other experiences were quite dire. The first time especially, after a boy turned me down. A boy who had serenaded me with a saxophone, kissed me, then apologized because he was seeing someone else. I ran back to my dorm in fumes that evening, and a friend suggested smoking to course correct the storm. To all our surprise, the "natural" substance that seems to pacify most people had an opposite effect on my temperament. Vacillating between cries and crackles of hysteria, my episode made for perpetual commentary among my dormmates.

The second time I smoked was with high school friends during winter break, barely able to breathe between excessive giggling. Yet after two emotionally draining "highs," I insisted on trying the ganja once again because Jennifer Martin is no quitter.

"Aren't you going to smoke with me?" I asked in Evan's Honda Civic as he parked between a cluster of cars. "Baby, you know I can't. It will

17

jeopardize my chance of getting into the FBI. Besides, one of us needs to stay sober." Evan said calmly as I rolled my eyes in the dark. *You're a college student, not a saint,* I thought. Between his accounting major, his political interests, and his dream of joining the FBI, I began wondering where I would stand between the edges of his projected goals. However, *I* never intended to apply for any job that requires a hair follicle drug screen, and eagerly exited the car for another chance to *do drugs*.

Evan and I tip-toed through the beer-soaked floors of the swim house and up to the attic. Slumped deep into their bean bags, three guys with blood-shot eyes remained tuned into their Mario Kart game, until the last racer fatefully fell off Rainbow Road and into infinity. The losing player dropped his controller, noticed me and Evan and asked: "Wanna hit?"

The calm stupor of my teammates seemed benign in contrast to the three-foot bong erected between the bean bags. Bongs had been an apparatus used by drug dealers in R-rated movies, yet here it was collecting resin IRL. I closed my gawking jaw and assured myself that drugs are cool and peer pressure is a challenge I welcome, then accepted their offer with grace. I bit down on my pride as my teammate offered fragmented instructions and held a lighter to the bowl. While I watched the smoke rise in the chamber, I took in a breath as deep as Michael Phelps.' As the vapor filled my lungs, I rejected the intake and started coughing incessantly, overhearing my teammates laugh in approval, patting my back and assuring me to not worry, that "coughing gets you higher."

And higher I flew throughout the next few hours. Unable to keep my composure while playing Nintendo, I asked Evan to escort me to a more isolated room. There, he held me as I silently delved deep into my repressed thoughts of food, fat, and failure. Every meal from the past month surfaced in my mind, making my head pound as I critiqued each slice of drunken pizza with disapproval. It was during this intoxicated stupor of high thoughts that

I knew I wanted - no, needed - to lose the few pounds I had put on during my first year, and that Ed had slipped back into my consciousness.

The rest of my "high" looked more like crying myself to sleep in Evan's arms after he drove me back to his apartment. He was stern, saying he didn't like how I reacted to pot, but acknowledged it was my choice if I were to keep smoking as summer approached. He protested, however, when he noticed the ink on my hand reading 'NO' one night at a house party.

"Jenny…" Evan said with disappointment as he lifted my scribbled hand to his face.

"It's not what you think it is." I said sheepishly.

I drew my hand away from his, ashamed for lying to the one person on campus that knew me best. I could lie about being at the library when I was running on the treadmill, or say I ate a sandwich for lunch when I only had an apple. But I could not hide this reminder to starve when I conspicuously tattooed the message on my skin.

With May drawing near, Evan largely brushed aside the matter. The semester was ending, and he aimed to savor our final weeks together on campus. Like any blooming romance, it was difficult to say our goodbyes as we parted for summer vacation. However, returning to Kansas City healed much of my heartache. Graduation parties celebrated my younger friends, and I was reunited with familiar faces. At one party, a mother of a long-time friend waved me down before she remarked: "You're supposed to *gain* weight in college!" At another party, an old teammate studying at NYU beamed as he told me I looked "New York Skinny." While I partially felt self-conscious from my apparent skeletal structure, I could hear Ed cheering me on from inside the compliment.

Comments about my size followed me like flies orbiting a picnic table, peaking during my lifeguard shifts at a neighborhood pool. Friends, teachers, and old high school crushes made frequent and candid observations about my 00 frame inside my two-piece lifeguard suit.

"Holy shit, I didn't notice you!" One person would say.

"Oh my god. You're so skinny. I'm so jealous." Another would comment.

"Damn Jen. I can see all your ribs."

I loved every moment of it. I loved lifting my shirt each morning to reveal the spaces between my rib cage, and witnessing my appetite shrivel day by day. A piece of fruit could sustain me between a morning workout and lunch, during which I ripped a bowl before taking the first bite. I had come a long way from my first few times getting high. Weed welcomed a better buzz than alcohol ever could and helped me tolerate the times I ate. Smoking made me hyper-aware of how my body felt. I could eat a little bit and embrace each bite as it slowly made its way down my system. By late June, I was a fully functioning anorexic stoner. My parents had no clue of my hippie habits, but they did express their concern about my weight frequently. "You're too skinny, Jenny!" cried my mom one day in the kitchen. Her eyes drilled through my bowed legs as I squirted mustard on canned tuna.

"Jesus, are we doing this again?" I thought as I took a breath to calm the energy in the room.

"Mom, I don't know what to say. I'm an athlete. I eat clean. I don't skip meals and I snack throughout the day. It's not like I'm not losing my hair or my period. You are overreacting." I slipped my mashed-up meal into a wrap of romaine, placating my mother's comment while I counted the calories of my lunch in my head, which added up to eighty.

"Jenny, *everyone* is talking about your weight loss. I hear it all the time. I talked to Evan. He's concerned for you, too."

With this intel, I dropped my wrap as my appetite withered away.

...

"My mom called you?" I asked Evan over the phone in fury.

"Jenny, she called out of love because she is concerned. We both love you and you know I think you're beautiful no matter your size."

"But why didn't you say something? I feel ambushed." I refuted.

"The timing didn't feel right. I want to see you happy, and I know this can be hard for you to hear. Just promise both of us that you'll try eating more." Evan said softly.

I paused before offering an obligatory "ok" in response. I could convince Evan over the phone, but I knew I wouldn't be able to convince myself of this empty promise. It didn't matter how many people told me they loved me or that I would still be beautiful if I gained weight, what mattered to me and what mattered to Ed was staying thin.

If beauty was power, then certainly skinny held power as well. Though the more weight I lost, the more I felt powerless to Ed's demands. I could hear a voice telling me, "This is wrong," right before Ed reminded me that "no one will want me in any other size." The summer stripped me away from any ambition beyond sharpening myself down to the bone, as my obsession with food became a part of my personality.

As sophomore year approached, I fancied the idea of being back on campus with my team and my boyfriend, away from the criticism in Kansas City. I didn't have an eating problem, but a problem with everyone at home commenting on my eating. However, Ed latched onto me like a leech, following me from state to state. My lack of muscle mass made practices drag on for what seemed like eternities. Though this intensive exercise had become my main driver keeping me on the team. Swimming turned into something to do to stay fit and feel like I belonged on campus, though Evan's absence at practice only dampened the situation.

Meanwhile, quitting the swim team turned out to be a greater burden for Evan than he expected. He felt increasingly isolated from his swimming roommates, and his self-doubt became a major turn-off. Our love became laced with aggravation, a feeling I preferred to hold at arm's length. So, instead of tending to Evan's needs, I preoccupied my thoughts on how to best constrict my food. When my parents drove up to see me again in October, my mom had nothing to say about my cheeks, as I deliberately worked to keep nothing in them.

The Monday after I said goodbye to my parents, my coach asked me into his office for a meeting.

"Hey, if this is about leaving early on Thursday's, it's because I'm required to take-"

"Oh, don't worry about your schedule. That's not what this is about." interrupted my coach. He seemed flustered.

"Jenny, your dad emailed me over the weekend to express his concern about your weight. I forwarded the message over to the school's trainer, and we've decided it's best we take careful measures to monitor your health. Tomorrow after practice, I'll take you to a sports nutritionist off campus. This is all for your wellbeing." He said without hesitation.

I nodded my head in compliance, attempting to hide my dismay before dashing out of his office to process what had just happened.

Dad?

Not Dad. He never got involved. He was supposed to be the one to scold me for buying beer with a fake ID, while Mom was the parent to pester me about my weight. I called my father after the meeting, asking for an explanation.

"Jenny, your mother and I love you." He paused, then persisted.

"We are only doing this because we care about you. I'm worried about your heart. That you're putting too much stress on it. You have a gene of addiction. My vices were drinking and drugging, and I'm afraid you're battling with food. You're the skinniest girl on your team, on any team. Your mother and I just want you to be strong again."

I gripped the phone to my ear, speechless. Choking back tears, I cleared my throat to respond.

"Yea. Yes. I'll try harder. I'll listen to the nutritionist and do whatever it takes to put on muscle." I said, trying hard not to cry and trying harder to believe that what I was saying was true. My coach and my parents were right. I was underweight, no doubt about that. But I could not grasp what was so wrong *about* my weight, as there were still soft parts of my stomach that I could pinch, that I wanted to go away.

For a moment, I held my promise to appease the adults. I ate larger portions and stopped running between practices. During the appointment with the sports nutritionist, we calculated my resting metabolic rate, which is the amount of calories a person burns in a day by simply existing. Turns out, I was eating about the same number of calories a day as I would burn from watching movies in bed. Realizing my two-a-day practices certainly allowed me to eat more, I became more accepting towards filling my plate. But as I tried to improve my relationship with food, my bond with Evan began to weaken.

During our one-year anniversary, I called things off between me and Evan. A "you don't have to plan anything special" for our date escalated into "I want to take a break." I could not help but feel that we were enabling each other's malaise, bound by a shared sense of melancholy. He loved me as much as he wanted my comfort, but I couldn't offer the support he sought from my brittle bones.

Evan and I had something special. We felt it. Our friends affirmed it. But sometimes passion - hell, true love - is not enough to bind two people. Possessiveness and passive-aggressive comments picked at the stitches holding our relationship together. He was a black suit dating a floral sundress that was a bit too short; our styles just didn't fit. Like fashion trends, our history was intense yet ephemeral. I truly did love him, and somewhere in my heart I always will. I will always think kindly of him, wishing him well, and hoping he forgives me for the turmoil I caused when lust led us back together.

Narcissistic Thoughts and Drunken Exclamations

"What's this?" My head cocked at the sight of the sheet. The paper was warm, fresh from the printer.

"This is your contract" snapped Jill, the university's head trainer. My coach asked me to meet him at Jill's office for an end-of-season meeting.

"What type of contract? Like for my scholarship?" I squinted my eyes towards Jill, then back to the pages in my hands. The college logo was stamped in the top right corner, with my name in the header. Everything below could have been written in hieroglyphics, as I was unable to decipher what the heck was going on.

"No, no. This is unique to your situation," said Jill.

"My situation?" I mumbled, fearing this concerned my weight.

"Your weight situation, Jennifer!"

I suddenly felt faint, but that could have been due to my 48-hour fruit cleanse. I might have also had a mild hangover from slapping a bag of wine the night before, which of course, counts as fruit.

"What does this mean? What do I need to do?" I asked, looking to my coach for comfort.

"In order to keep your scholarship, we're asking you to maintain a healthy weight." My coach chimed in, wearing a collar whiter than the wall he leaned up against, his face one shade warmer.

"Which is...?" *Which is the most important detail of this conversation.*

"120 pounds. We'll have you come in for weekly weigh-ins to record your progress and if the weight isn't met, you'll be put on athletic probation." Jill answered, stiff as her clipboard which held her copy of the contract.

One hundred and twenty pounds! Those three numbers expanded in my mind's eye like fireworks in the night, malfunctioning into mayhem. 120 was burned and branded into my brain.

1-2-0. Alongside this astronomical number was a whining Ed, throwing a hissy fit in my hippocampus.

Jill handed me a pen to sign the document. She might as well have handed me an ink-blotted dumbbell.

"Thank you, Jennifer. We will see you in August. Have a nice summer." Jill nodded and exited out to the training room.

I looked over to my coach like a dog watching their owner grab their coat, but not the leash. Soon, I would be gone for the summer, left to my own devices. And by no means was I an essential swimmer to the team - it's not like I was winning us titles and breaking records. But I was a part of the team - a part of his program. But I was falling apart and letting everyone down.

"Take care of yourself, Jenny." My coach led me to the hallway and gave me a hug.

"Thank you." I sighed as the conversation started to settle. Perhaps it was time to finally comply with the adults' requests and trust that they knew what was in my best interest. Perhaps it was time to surrender and sever ties with Ed.

...

My twentieth birthday was approaching, and I weighed the same as when I was thirteen. While shaking my bony ass to "Headlines" and other Drake songs one afternoon in my bathroom, I dusted bronzer to further define my cheeks and highlight my bulging collarbones. All vibes were high until I slid down the stairs to find my parents gatekeeping the garage. My buzz now fizzled into paranoia. Suspicions suspended in the air. Clearly, I had been the topic of a recent conversation.

"What?" I asked defensively.

"Jenny, have a seat," said my dad. He meant at the dinner table, but I plopped on the staircase to keep higher ground.

"Have you been purging?" He asked.

My heart pounded in my chest, enraged at the accusation. It had been a month since signing the contract concerning my weight, providing plenty of time for me to pack on a couple pounds before the fall semester. Though that June I slipped back into restrictive diets and obsessive exercising, prancing around in swimsuits or sports bras, wearing little with nothing to hide. Skin stuck to my bones like sealant, wrapping tightly around every sharp edge of my frame.

"You hardly fit into your clothes!" My mom yelled. I stood up and stepped down to my parent's level, rolling my eyes while explaining "it's a *shift dress*."

My arms crossed stiff against my ribs as I fumed in the kitchen. After all, it was my 20th birthday. I was expecting a card, not an intervention.

"No! I'm not puking, Dad. I eat healthy, I work out. I'm a college athlete, of course I'm going to be thin!" I shouted. How dare they suggest such a ravenous act. I was *anorexic*. Bulimia, however, was not a territory I had crossed... *Yet.*

My mom held her head in her hands, "but you are *too* thin, Jenny. Everyone thinks so."

Does everyone think so? I trembled in my XS dress at 5 feet, 7 inches, 118 pounds and 17 percent body fat. I surveyed these statistics every day that summer, as the 120-pound burden etched into my thoughts.

Two pounds. Only two pounds. I told myself to sustain 118 over the summer before I faced the scale in August. *But I don't want to gain two pounds. I like the way I look and the attention I receive around my thinness.* This was my first summer in college as an independent woman, where I was free to flirt vivaciously in little clothing, revealing all. My parents saw my frail limbs as a sign of an eating disorder, but I saw them as an achievement.

For me, restriction was a sport. Surviving on less calories than the day before affirmed that I could live off so little. Though little was I aware of what voids I devised inside from this saga of starvation.

To an outsider, I was considered lucky. Young, attractive, physically inclined, and smart enough to maintain an academic scholarship without trying too hard. Afterall, the scant glucose fueling my brain was used for calculating the amount of glucose I was consuming. To an outsider, I was considered popular. Bubbly and bouncing between social circles. I knew a lot of people, but no one knew the real me. I didn't know the real me. But I was pretty good at looking pretty and distracting myself with peers who could drink and smoke weed like me. Friendships came easily, yet sporadically. Like my friendship with Alyssa, which ebbed and flowed further and further away. As she took summer courses, I studied nutrition labels and tested out which bars would accept my fake ID. Though at 20 years old, I realized one day I would pop out of the campus bubble to work in the real world. This concerned me. How would my pretty, party-girl persona survive in a corporate office?

The rest of the summer dragged on as I ran through heat waves between my summer job as a swim coach at Indian Hills Country Club. Located in Kansas City's wealthiest neighborhood, Indian Hills has a vastly different appeal than Brookridge, the club my family belonged to in an area with a quarter of the market value. Indian Hills upholds a culture of inheritance, reputation, and esteemed image. Moms watched me coach in my one-piece and swooned over my small frame in their Tory Burch sandals. They would pick up Savanna and Chandler after a Pilates class decked in Lululemon, peer through their Chanel sunglasses and gasp, "Wow, Jenny. I'd kill to have your body." Those compliments were my nutrition as I fed off their influence, hoping one day I would end up like one of them: an affluent trophy wife with the self-control to stay perpetually petite.

As for my parents, they were not concerned with the ranking of their club so long as they could play golf. My dad grew up not too far from Indian Hills, in a simple, three-bedroom house with strict, Catholic parents and his six siblings. He attended high school amongst his rich peers and started working as a golf caddy for their rich parents. This motivated him to lead a life of leisure for himself, and through decades of working the 12-Steps of AA and climbing a few corporate ladders, he eventually retired with enough cash to purchase a condo down in Florida where he snowbirds in the winter. Not a bad life, considering how before he got sober, he "didn't have a pot to piss in."

Today, when I visit my dad in the sunshine state, we drive through subdivisions of million-dollar mansions along the gulf coast while listening to classic rock.

"Who sings this?" He asks in his Genesis.

"The Eagles." I say, reading credits off the dashboard.

We then pass a home as vast as Hotel California, where my dad points at an iron gate and remarks: "all you have to have is money."

My mother, a frugal gal, feels most comfortable spending her money at the Home Depot. The flashiest item in her closet is a small Coach purse I insisted she buy, only so I could borrow it. She grew up comfortably in St. Louis with smart, sensible, loving parents, and showed the same amount of care to me and Matt. When my mom wasn't working as a nurse, she was taking my brother and I to various practices, repairing *everything* around the house all while cooking, cleaning, reading for bible study and of course, playing golf. Always active, my mom hardly visited the gym. She rarely wore makeup, saying how it is not as important as wearing a smile. She puts her fork down when she is full, never shaming herself for what was on her plate. And never, *ever* in my upbringing did I hear her comment on her weight.

However, for me, what I ate and how much I weighed was all my mom and dad could talk about that summer when I turned twenty-one. Thus, pacifying their concern became my full-time job. I picked meals and mealtimes strategically; eating little at Indian Hills and mostly at home when my parents were present. But as much as I talked about food in front of my parents, cooked and baked and ate in front of my parents, my attempts to look like I was adequately eating were not fooling anyone. They were only deceiving me.

Mid-August approached, commencing junior year and an escape from parental pressures. Though before we parted ways, my mom and dad helped me to settle into my new place just one block off campus. I was one of four girls who would soon be living in frat-house conditions with a feminine touch. Mismatched furniture covered (some of) the carpet stains, but we pulled the living room together with a collection of acrylics I painted as a project to ignore my appetite while getting stoned. I peppered the canvases along moldy walls of a house I was ready to call home.

As my parents and I assembled furniture upstairs in my room, I heard the laugh of my roommate and teammate, Carly.

"JENNY!" She jumped through the door, giggled, and gave me a tight squeeze. Carly was an Ohio native, an education major and force of positivity. She has that kind of vibrant laugh that naturally inclines you to laugh with her. Carly leaned back from our hug and scanned me, head to toe.

"You've gotten stronger!" she exclaimed as she grabbed my bicep.

Right. In front. Of my parents.

I felt relieved, overjoyed, and confident in entering this new year and leaving the parental stress of the summer behind.

Then my other roommate, Lilly, burst into the room to welcome me home. As I reached around her for a hug, the cold condensation of a Smirnoff Ice bottle damped her back underneath her sports bra.

"Gotcha, Jenny! You've been *iced.*"

My parents rolled their eyes as I took a knee and proceeded with a couple chugs of sparkling malt liquor.

"To education!" I cheered.

Unimpressed, my mom and dad shooed us downstairs so they could finish setting up my bed without distraction. God bless syllabus week; it truly is the most wonderful time of the year.

It wouldn't be a stretch to say that I remained buzzed throughout that entire first week back at school. There were simply too many people to see, parties to attend, and freshmen to kiss. I didn't have time to be sober. I didn't make time to eat. Suddenly it was Friday. It was time to weigh in.

Oh shit.

I found myself lined up with my teammates outside the training room, where our university's name stretched across the wall. One by one, Jill the trainer summoned the swimmers in for a physical.

Shit. shit. shit.

I had sweat off at least a pound under the midday sun during yesterday's dryland workout and could feel another pound shed as I trembled in my tracksuit, fearing the number about to appear under my toes.

"118.8"

Shit, shit, NO!

My head hung low as I stepped off the scale, lifting only to catch Jill's reaction. I waited for her to pause this standard procedure and announce to the team my immediate probation. But nothing happened. Jill stoically took my figures and waved over the next girl.

I bolted home after the physical; it was only a matter of time before my Blackberry beeped with an email from the training office. As each hour passed without a notification, I figured I was not a significant enough asset to the team to warrant attention. Though by 9pm that Friday night, I was less concerned about my athletic career and fully invested in planning a string of festivities.

While casting out texts, I sipped on a Smirnoff Ice and considered my disposition as a student athlete. Every day, we work out together, eat together, and study together. Then, we party and sleep together. The swimcest epidemic is a real thing amongst campuses. Some baseball boys even called us a cult. Such homogeneous relations apply to all coed teams, without having a ring to the disturbing name: *swimcest*.

Though my loyalty to the team was declining, I felt obligated to start the night with my fellow swimmers. Besides, none of my normie friends were getting back to me with plans. I soon gathered around a makeshift beer-pong table with my roommates and a couple of sophomores in the communal area of a dorm, eagerly double-texting my non-swimmer pals. A soft murmur filled the room as the other girls checked a message I had not received.

"What's up gang? Where are the party people headed to tonight?" I asked my younger teammates in a patronizing tone.

"Um… everyone is going to Evan's house tonight." A sophomore, Jamie, said sheepishly.

"O really! *How fun.*" I bit my tongue, resisting the upchuck from that unsettling news.

Evan quit the team over a year ago. He was a senior now and had moved into a* NARP house. *(Non-Athletic-Regular-People). Why would he invite the team - *the freshmen* - to get piss drunk at his house? Clearly, this was a trap. Obviously, this was about me.

Carly noticed my disappointment and came over to console me. "We can go home together if you want. I don't have to go out."

I contemplated her offer, considering how appealing a bowl of weed in bed sounded and my lack of alternative plans. "You guys go, I'll text some people…. don't worry about me." I sighed.

"No, no, Jenny just come. A ton of people will be there, you won't run into him." Jamie intervened and you know what, Jamie was right. What were the chances Evan would notice his ex-girlfriend traverse his humble abode among a sea of swimmers?

I grabbed a bottle of cherry vodka, along with Jamie and a freshman. We split the remains of the bottle as I led the girls out the dorm down to the street, preaching all the way to the party.

"Ladieees. Let me set some ground rules for college. Mm kay? Rule nummer one, don't date swimmers, you'll break up and he'll invite all your friends to his party, and it will be awkward. Rule nummer two, make friends outside the swim team. Swimmers are overrated and you'll get sick of partying with them. And nummer three. This is impornan! Always, *always* leave a full water bottle by your bed before you go out."

I stopped to check that my young proteges were paying attention.

"Most importan ruuule- are yew listening? Don't date swimmers. The swim team sucks."

"But don worry… College is awesome. YOLO."

I got so wrapped up in counseling my newest teammates that we nearly walked past Evan's house, which would have been such a shame!

I stared at Evan's porch from the sidewalk as Carly and Lilly caught up with the migrating swim team. The front door was propped open. Ceiling lights illuminated every room. I could make out familiar faces as their laughter mocked me from the outside. When I was told the swim team was invited, it was inferred that the extension was not meant to reach me.

"Are you sure you want to go inside? We can head back right now, really, it's not a big deal" Carly protested.

"No, it's fine" I shot back. "I'm drunk, it's like, whatever. Let's go."

A faint scent of nostalgia and regret stalled in the foyer. I entered the inevitable quagmire with a confident yet sleepy smile, hiding my inner turmoil of the impending discomfort. I couldn't socialize alone and appointed my girlfriends as bodyguards. I also couldn't stand up straight, so they escorted me to the couch in the crowded living room. Sinking into the cushion, I pretended that I never caught a glimpse of Evan in the kitchen. I pretended that I couldn't see him watching me out of the corner of my heavy eyes. I pretended that he wasn't walking up to me from the beer pong table.

Wait, no, he was headed straight towards me. The next thing I knew, he was holding my hand and leading me towards the door. Someone started to play Taylor Swift's *"I Knew You Were Trouble"* on full blast from the speakers.

Confused, I kept quiet and complied, taking Evan's hand as he ushered me down the sidewalk. I pressed my body close to his. A feeling of safety reverberated off his chest. My head kept close to his neck as I whispered "I'm sorry" in his ear.

Approaching my place, Evan swept my keys from my little lime green crossbody and guided me into my room. He laid me down on top of my bed with no intention of joining. I could not grasp why he had come so far only to drift away. I grabbed onto his hand, widened my sleepy eyes, and pouted my lips, chanting:

"But I love you." I begged as Evan tucked me under my sheets.

"Tell me that in the morning, then we can talk" he said as he shut my door behind him.

An alarm blared by my head. I blindly patted my dresser for my phone, fighting to gain consciousness.

SMS TEXT:

11:58 PM Ally C: Did Evan go home with u last night?!?

This message from Ally, my old roommate slash teammate slash former BFF confirmed everything I was trying to piece back together. Ally was my first roommate, whom I drew a mutual affection towards during the dawn of college. Though when I started dating Evan, my friendship with Ally took a turn as I directed much time and attention towards my boyfriend. And while I did not turn away from my gal pals completely, I was unable to manage expectations with Ally. We eventually realized that I cannot cap myself with one "bestie" or a particular "girl gang." By our junior year, we came to a cordial dynamic as party friends and shared a mutual apathy towards the swim team. Ally and I bonded over our boredom with the sport and created countdowns from syllabus week until the end of the season. We were now homies but not besties. That junior year, I spent a considerate amount of time at Ally's, who happened to live next door to Evan.

Evan.

A flood of emotions supercharged my hangover as I burrowed in bed, drowned by thoughts of Evan swirling in my head. I loved Evan, but I could not be with him. I wanted to support him, but I could not date him. I knew Evan could give me what I needed emotionally, but I would no longer be able to reciprocate.

Evan was two semesters away from stepping foot into "the real world," a place which I was in no rush to visit. He was already interning with the city mayor and enrolling into graduate school, whereas I piled on pass-fail classes and sought out loopholes in my (now communications) major. The plan was to jam my junior year with credits so I could coast by as a senior and still walk out with a diploma.

Evan was maturing into a fine gentleman of society, and I was looking to get laid. And with that intention, I went out and did just that with a man we will call Jack. Jack was a transfer student on the baseball team; tall, dark, handsome and within minutes of meeting him, wooed by my beer pong skills and endearing, tipsy charm. Though when the booze wore off, so did the excitement. My ardent attempts to be a "cool girl" seemed to freeze over the heat between us two after our third hook-up, when he started dating a soccer player who showed more promise of girlfriend material.

A week after me and the baseball boy simmered, I struck out again with a man I had been crushing on since day one of college. Let's call him Joe. This dude led me on throughout freshman orientation only to admit he was seeing someone else when tension peaked. Joe was the guy who serenaded me with his saxophone, bought me a turkey sandwich at Subway, and dropped the ball on his unavailable status after kissing my cheek. This collision of mixed signals propelled me into a spiral when I picked up weed for the first time. Months later while dating Evan, Joe reached out to be all, "I noticed you're dating and I'm dating and I'm so happy to see you happy," which made me happy, and we remained friends. As the years passed and my relationship with Evan dwindled, Joe started showing extra interest in our friendship. We remained so friendly, in fact, that by junior year Joe consistently smoked me up after partying, often inviting me to spend the night. Golly! What a nice guy.

It was now late September and everyone on campus sensed this would be the last hot weekend of the summer. Better make it count by making the hemlines short. I slipped into a flaming red dress, the kind that makes you hard to ignore and even harder to sit down. But I managed to sit before responding to Joe's text and drank a Smirnoff Ice while Lilly curled my hair.

"It's going to happen tonight," I told Lilly.

"How do you know?" she asked while the iron warmed my skull. I paused and laughed at all of Joe's advancements. I stared at Lilly in the mirror and replied, "the dress."

I made up my mind. I was going home with Joe.

And I did. We intersected during a string of party hopping and bounced back to his 100-year-old, six-bedroom house he shared with five other rugby players. Ah, rugby players. The sex was steamy and drunk and recurred every few hours like clockwork. We cuddled in between, talking about his travel stories and plans for law school, and my managing a social life as a student athlete. By noon the next day, we both agreed it was time to disperse and study. Joe handed me clothes to change into, took me home in his black sedan and kissed me on my driveway.

"You're impressive, Jenny," Joe said.

I gave him another kiss and stepped out of the car.

"Thank you" I said smiling, feeling very impressive indeed.

But on Monday, I was not so impressed when Joe never reached out. On Tuesday, I kindly reminded Joe about his clothes and when I could return them.

SMS TEXT:

10:38 AM: JENNY: Hey you. I have some fresh laundry for ya. When can I come by?

3:38 PM: JOE: Hey Jenny. I'm still getting over a breakup. I just don't think I'm ready to see people right now.

The earth rippled beneath me as I shook from this shift. I thought I held the power in this game. I thought I had the final say in this play.

I spent that night sulking in my room, contemplating how I would surely die alone, survived by a beta fish and dehydrated plants in a Midwestern apartment.

Then my Blackberry beeped. My long-awaited email popped on the screen. Jill the trainer sent a short notification that excused me from practice that week. I'd been put on probation.

Heartache morphed into rage and worry as I registered the email. A month had passed since the initial weigh-in, and from my increased intake of booze, I had undoubtedly reached 120 lbs. I was to weigh in on Thursday morning for another assessment. To be safe on the scale, I called a NARP friend to join me for a beer... or eight.

This friend, Margaret, was a fun time to be around, if and when she was ever around. Not necessarily a reliable friend, I knew I could count on her to get excessively drunk with me on a Wednesday night.

Amusingly Margaret lived with Ally, who lived across from Evan. Therefore, every time I hung out with Margaret, I had the pleasure of walking past Evan's house, hoping that he was elsewhere. And while Evan never had nice things to say about Margaret while we were dating, he became partial to Margaret that year as neighbors.

"Evan just asked if I wanted to come over to finish a keg" Margaret said as she twirled her curly black hair.

"He said to invite whoever." She added while investigating a possible split end.

"Does he know I'm with you?" I asked.

"Oh yea. He knows you're with me." Margaret brushed her hair away and handed me a bottle of cherry vodka to pull back before walking next door. There, Evan answered in a fitted gray sweater, showing off the tone in his arms he had noticeably gained since our breakup. He led us towards the keg in the kitchen, where I sipped on my foamy Solo cup, observing Evan as he observed me. He looked like such a man. He spoke in a sophisticated, grown-up, man-like way. While he ranted about Ohio democrats, I smiled at him in adoration to both flirt with wide eyes and conceal my lack of understanding or care about the subject at hand.

After another diluted beer, my wide eyes became real tough to keep open, and I called it a night. Evan walked me to the front door, all calm and coy. His body language vetoed any initiation for a hug, so I held his face in a mental snapshot, hoping next time I'd be able to hold his head in my hands.

Hours later, a familiar alarm penetrated through my bedroom walls. By reflex, I got up to change for practice, only to remember that I could not attend. Exclusion guarded my door, warning me to stay in bed while I listened to my roommate's drawers slide open and close. I once dreamt of the day I'd hit REM sleep at 5am rather than hitting snooze, and now that this day had come, I felt like I was cheating myself of something. All my life I was "Jenny the swimmer." I didn't know how to just be Jenny. Swimming brought belonging and gave me an edge - beyond the sharp corners of my shoulders, hips, and knees. How would people know my name if it wasn't embroidered on a varsity jacket? And what about my workouts? Would I be able to maintain my physique without a coach and a team to train with? Such questions haunted me as I fell back asleep.

Once my alarm went off at 7am, I raced to the cafeteria before any of my teammates would see me after practice. I had an hour to chow down before my weigh-in. I first scoured the selection of pastries - an area of the mess hall I typically eschewed. My eyes burned from the light reflecting off the crystal glaze of a Danish, frosted with enough sugar to tamper the scale. But one Danish would not do the trick, I needed sustenance. I needed savory. So, I plucked the pastry from the display to my tray and darted down the line for cheesy scrambled eggs. Next to my pile of yellow goop, I plopped a couple scoops of crispy, golden tater tots. Add a few pumps of scarlet corn syrup from the Heinz dispenser, and baby girl is set. I found an inconspicuous corner to drop off my tray, then made way to the chocolate milk dispenser to help wash this feast down.

Walking back towards my solitary booth, the tray glowed like Aztec Gold, with my gaze as feral as Jack Sparrow. I grabbed my fork and started digging. Mouth salivating, mind exploding. Bud and booze couldn't compete with the relief of fried spuds and melted cheese. I hadn't felt this high since my first time rolling MDMA the previous spring. My dopamine receptors couldn't tell the difference between a rave and a doughnut, but my taste buds were relieved considering molly tastes like ass. Then Ed sat down beside me. *"That's enough. It's time to go."*

I wobbled across campus, frazzled and ashamed. The glass doors to the training room seemed heavier than usual. The hallway was bright and sterile. But not me - I tracked mud from all my dirty deeds. You could smell my misconduct from across the room and Jill wasted no time for bullshit.

"Step on," Jill motioned towards the scale. Fortunately, I did not recognize any athletes in the room receiving physical therapy. I shook off my sneakers and stepped on the smooth metal plate, watching the digits dance as they calculated my weight.

121.1 lbs.

Idiots. You happy now?

"Cool. Can I go back to practice?" I asked super-duper maturely.

"Not quite. You'll have to train on your own until your probation is cleared, which will take a couple more signatures. Your contract continues until the end of the year, but your weekly weigh-ins will now be with a physician in the university health center. Which is where your psychologist, Dr. Lacy, will meet you twice a month." Jill responded and motioned to the door.

I was *livid*. On top of my 18-hour course load, two-a-day practices and partying, I now had mandated visits to the health center. For what? I weighed 121.1 lbs. for Pete's sake!

Steam evaporated off my head in the crisp fall air as I walked to the rec center to practice on my own. Luckily at this hour, hot Chad was lifeguarding the pool, so I took my time fidgeting with my goggles while standing on the gutter. Chad was a close friend of Evan, Margaret, and by default, me. But our dynamic convoluted that semester each afternoon we smoked weed together, escalating after he wrote a Theology paper for me.

Twenty-five yards away, I waved down my dark-eyed friend as I stood half-naked on the deck. I strapped on my cap and goggles and dove into my desolate lane, paddling through the water in solace of my solitude. Without any coaches to keep me accountable, I took my time on sets and skipped intervals to flirt with the lifeguard.

"Hey Chad. You bored?" I asked knowing he was both stoned and indubitably bored.

"Hey Jen. Why aren't you practicing with the team?"

I gazed down the gutter, "It's a long story, but let's just say my schedule cleared up this week."

"Sweet. Well, hit me up when you're free." Chad nodded.

A tingling came over me. Chad suddenly looked more buff than usual. I gulped an inhale and sunk into the water, diluting my thoughts from the gutter. I couldn't hook up with Chad. He was Evan's best friend! That would be *fucked up*.

I tried to trail out of the locker room before the rest of my team arrived for afternoon practice, but I couldn't sneak past the pool rats. Just as I locked up, my team captains, Heather and Kayla, strolled into the scene.

"Jenny... we heard what happened." Heather said as she peered into my face, scanning for answers around my absence.

I diverted my eyes from hers, alluding to her intel that something had *"happened."*

"How much training will you miss?" asked Kayla as she applied athletic tape to her shoulder.

Please, princess.... Don't act like you haven't missed any practices over the past three years due to your recurring injuries.

"Oh, hey guys. I'm great. I'll be in the pool with everyone soon. I'd love to chat, but I have homework." I lied.

I didn't have homework. I didn't *do* homework. Instead, I had therapy.

Dr. Lacy's office was stale. Gray as the sky in January and wide enough to fit her desk, the small bookcase behind it, and our two chairs. I wondered if Doc had any say over the decor, as the only thing hanging on the wall was her PhD. Adjacent to her credentials was a small window, shining a halo over her strawberry blonde head.

"Why do you think you're here, Jenny?" Dr. Lacy asked after the introductory, *'tell me about yourself.'*

There was no need to schmooze Dr. Lacy, so I got to the point.

"I think my parents are worried about me. And I get it. I had moments where I was hyper-focused on eating healthy foods, and not eating enough calories as an athlete... Though I'm eating a lot more, honestly. And since my second weigh-in, I've stayed over 120 pounds."

I stopped there. I could see why last year's lowest weight at 114 was problematic and potentially lethal if I continued to drop. But I could not pinpoint *why* I wanted to drop and drop and drop.

"How have things changed this year?" She asked.

I flipped through every fragmental difference of junior year: I was now living off campus, maxed out in credit hours, crossing campus for weekly weigh-ins, classes, and practices all by foot. I hardly slept and was sleeping around. I was no longer with Evan.

"I'm single." I stared at the spines of Dr. Lacy's book collection, wondering how well she was about to read me.

"Tell me a little about that." Dr. Lacy asked, inducing relief. For once, the therapist did not ask me to elaborate over food.

"Evan, my first love, my first... *everything* and I split up before summer break. It was my decision, and while I still care about him, things wore off between us and I ultimately fell out of love." Phew, that came out so *easily*.

"How was your eating when you two were together?" She asked. Stumped, I recognized that my lowest weight occurred while dating Evan, but I had not considered the parallels between him and my other partner, Ed.

"Well, I ate more when I was around him, eating off his plate or sharing a cookie... things like that. But I guess I was more restrictive all around compared to how I've been eating this year."

"How did this affect the relationship?" Dr. Lacy asked.

I paused, considering the question in another light. I had thought my dainty frame validated our love, or at least my ability to receive it.

"Evan and I loved each other, and he wanted what was best for my health. And I knew that of all the people who have told me, 'Oh, you're beautiful no matter your size," Evan would surely still love me if I gained some weight. But I don't know... I still wanted to be thin for him." I melted into the cobalt couch, letting my words sink in. Dr. Lacy let me ponder for a while. My mind floated on a sea of reasoning above the bedrocks of control. Her next question shot me right back to reality.

"What does thinness mean to you?"

Approval. Acceptance. Marriage. I associated a lean frame with carats on a scrawny finger. But I did not dare say that aloud. Like any first love, I imagined marriage with Evan, until our differences blurred the dream. The futility of my disease evinced that I still had so much to see and do and learn about myself, the world, and relationships before any lifelong commitment.

"I guess it means beauty, right? All the magazines and Spice Girls and movies I watched made an impact." I sighed, relieved to admit that the desire to control my weight had multiple external influences. Couldn't we just blame Carrie Bradshaw and call it a day?

"Of course, Jenny. Your environment has a major impact on how you develop self-image, I am glad you see that." Dr. Lacy closed her notebook. "As you continue to build self-awareness, I encourage you to write down these realizations in a journal, if you don't already do so. Be completely honest with yourself in how you are feeling and eating. Call me if you need anything." Our time ended and while I had some resistance going into the meeting, I left feeling lighter. Not like, thinner lighter, but I felt less pressure to be so damn perfect. Her suggestion to journal was something I had done to count calories and meal plan in the past, but I was open to amending my entries. When I pulled out my phone to schedule our next appointment, my screen flashed a message from Chad.

SMS TEXT:

4:02 Chad M: It's almost that time – are you coming over?

At 4:02 PM, it was almost that time indeed. I booked my next visit with Dr. Lacy and skipped over to Chad's with eighteen minutes to spare. It was Thursday afternoon. Which in September, means a Thirsty Thursday for the swim team as competitions were weeks away. The men's team was hosting a house party, to which I showed up a little drunk and really stoned. (Chad's blunt really did me in). When I spotted Evan by the DJ table, I raced to the kitchen and ramped up my liquor intake. I tried avoiding the topic of my ex-boyfriend lingering in the premises, until Ally stepped into the room, stared at me with her ice blue eyes and asked:

"Jenny… Evan just put on Dave Matthews. Isn't that what you used to fuck to?" Ally cooed in my ear.

Playing Cupid, Ally planted seeds of sexual scenes into my head. I watered those seeds with bottom-shelf vodka to grow this idea that Evan was signaling me through nostalgia. Because yes, we used to fuck to the Dave Matthews Band, in proper millennial fashion. As "Tripping Billies" turned on, so did my libido. Hours passed as I waited for the crowd of swimmers to clear out, catching Evan in a private moment so the two of us could once again *"eat, drink, and be merry…"*

Then it happened. I woke up in Evan's arms, but in a different room. In a different bed. And while the eyes I stared into were familiar, I spoke to a different man. Gone was the boy filled with optimism and playful banter. No longer was I free to be myself around the person I used to love.

I rolled towards him, about to reach around for his firm, bare waist. "As much as I'm sure you're relieved to sleep in, I'm afraid I have to get ready for work." Evan said quickly as he pushed my hand away.

Before I could hold him, press my nose into his shoulder and squeeze him one more time, I retracted flat on my back. My eyes glared at the ceiling, too embarrassed to look elsewhere.

"Here, drink some water, Jen." Evan motioned with a glass waving above my head.

I grabbed the bed sheets to cover my chest as I curled up against the headboard, relieved to be drinking something that wasn't alcohol.

"Thank you." I said looking into the glass, waiting for the water to forecast the subsequent scenes like a crystal ball.

"You alright?" Evan asked. His tone was slightly condescending.

I went mute. *Was I alright?* I had just slept with a man I cared deeply about, yet no longer cared to be in a relationship with. Last night's pow-wow was fueled by a desperation for familiarity, closure, and of course, attention. If I could hop in his bed, maybe I would stay in his mind.

"Fine," I mumbled.

"You drank a lot last night." Evan said, oh so matter of fact.

"Thirsty Thursday." I shrugged.

Evan looked at me with disappointment. "You should get going."

Despite our history, this began to feel like another one-night-stand. As I gathered my clothes, I waited for my lover to offer me a ride back to my house, but nothing happened. How foolish of me, to think I deserved such a chivalrous gesture after treating him like dispensable commonfolk.

"Don't worry about leaving the door unlocked when you leave." Evan noted.

I walked home in yesterday's clothes and fading makeup ashamed and confused. I certainly didn't want a relationship with Evan, just his respect. Or at least, that's what I told myself. But I was seeking closure in his bed through casual sex, without paving room for intimacy. I wanted to make sure I was still lovable, and assessed that theory on my ex.

As I slipped into my 10:30 AM Communications class with seconds to spare, I felt my pocket buzz with a text from the same person sitting directly in front of me.

SMS TEXT:

10:28 AM Ally C: Did I hear "Crash Into Me" from next door last night, or was that just me?

My eyes rolled away from the white board, now glued to my screen. It didn't take a genius to see why my grades were slipping, as my mind primarily fixated on primal needs: food & sex. While my professor outlined press releases, I thought about pressing my body against another shirtless, sculpted chest.

To get my mind off men, I turned to the kitchen after class to do what anorexics do best: cook for other people. Though I wouldn't call myself Giada, I do a mean job of following a baking recipe. For a teammate's birthday, I prepared a spread of brownies and Cherry Jell-O shots, two treats that pair well with malt liquor. I offered these delicacies at a pregame party with the girls that Saturday night with the intent to win over the affection of the teammates I had deserted over the past few practices.

The brownies were a hit, but the Jell-O shots did not seem to win over the crowd. This was upsetting because dammit, I paid good money for that handle of McCormick's! I took this failure personally and started pressuring my peers, taking one shot for every three girls I convinced to join me. To put that number in perspective: Eighteen shots, divided by three, plus two cups of jungle juice taken by a 121.1 Lb. female… That's proper drunk. But since alcohol digests slower with Jell-O, I didn't feel as buzzed as I wanted to be in case I ran into Evan that night. To armor up, I jacked a Pabst from the fridge and chugged it in the bathroom, sitting on the toilet lid to drink in silence. I tilted my head back to shake out the last drops and crushed the can in my hand. I closed my eyes, licking the lager from my lips and savoring the darkness. My eyelids quivered as I tried opening them. My vision focused on a purple ceiling fan. My body… was horizontal. My face… was pressed against a sheet. My dress… was nowhere near my body.

I tucked my chin and gazed down at my chest. The yellow racerback tank that covered my top half was on backwards, exposing a nipple. As for downstairs, I bared all. Shivering in the fetal position, a blanket by my toes had fallen off to unveil my butt and (just one) boob.

I sensed a body next to mine, but I was too afraid to look over and see who it belonged to. It took every bit of energy and a gulp of pride for me to roll over and identify.

Hair. Long hair. Woman. Thank god it's a woman. Is that? Why yes, it's Margaret. We are all good people!

"Jeeeeenny" Margaret whispered as she turned to face me, her eyes still shut.

"You're alive!" She giggled.

Suddenly, Ally poked her blonde head through the bedroom door. "Jenny's alive!"

"Dude, you were puking red last night. Are you sure you're alive?" Ally asked.

Puking red? Damn, Jell-O shots will get you every time.

"I'm alive." I sighed in disbelief.

"And I blacked out."

Not that I thought blacking out was "cool," it seemed like a lot of people I considered cool at the time had cool stories of when they had done so. That is, drinking until the point of amnesia. With my dad being an alcoholic, I feared the black out as that seemed pretty alcoholic, and I surely didn't want to turn into no sweaty, red-faced alcoholic. I just wanted to drink excessively without consequences.

There's a crude joke on a T-shirt you can find in the average Barstool bro's closet that says, "My drinking team has a (swimming) problem", with swimming being an interchangeable verb. As much as I wanted to avoid the stigma of alcoholism, there was an underlying implication that if you swam, you drank. And drink we did.

Hours after leaving Margaret's, I made it back to my own bed, with my own clothes, worn the right way.

BING!

It was an email from Jill. I was cleared from probation and would presume practices with the team first thing Monday morning.

Well, this was... good news? NGL, I was starting to get used to NARP life. Sleeping in and sleeping around made me feel like a regular

47

college kid. But then again, I didn't want to be regular. So, I jumped back into my regularly scheduled programming.

Suddenly, it was Thursday. Who's Thirsty?

Remember Chad? Hot Chad? The lifeguard I asked to write my theology paper for me? Of course you do. What type of sick person exchanges drugs for plagiarized literature on morals and ethics? *This girl.*

I arrived at Chad's apartment with a bottle of UV Blue in hand and an intention to "brown" out. (Blacking out was now reserved for Saturdays when I didn't have practice the next morning). Chad, Margaret, and Chad's roommate Curtis were inside, violently hitting the hued vodka I had provided. Amid playing a round of non-strategic drinking games, Curtis blurted out: "Hey Jenny, since Chad wrote your paper… you're going to have to repay him with some favors. You know which favors I'm talking about."

Whereas some people lose their filter when drinking, Curtis was born without one. He saw the tension building between me and Chad and tersely pointed it out. My flushed cheeks, increased heart rate and perspiration were normal vital changes from alcohol, but any sober person could tell you that these were direct effects of affection for a particular person in that room.

I smiled at Curtis and winked at Chad. "No worries, Curtis, it's all been taken care of." We all took one more pull of the UV Blue and headed to a house party.

Chad and I took a cab home early, leaving the party faster than I could pull off my top. I gripped onto Chad's shoulders as I leaned down to kiss him. My knees clamped his torso as my lips pressed against his. I reached for his belt.

"No, Jenny… we can't. Evan's my friend"

I pulled my head back and pressed my hand on his chest, replying "so?" with my eyes.

"But you're so pretty," Chad sighed.

I squeezed his hip, and he let out a quiet "*fuck.*"

We kept things mostly PG and above the pants, though this hookup was for mature audiences only. Only, neither of us were that mature ourselves. Just two twenty-year-olds akin by sexual build up and stamina.

Not much later, my alarm went off on Chad's desk. We woke up both fully clothed in his twin bed with my body pinned up against the wall.

"Shit. I have practice." I moaned.

"Here," Chad motioned to his keys.

"Take my car to the rec center. I can walk to work."

Woah, Chad just trusted me with his keys. He must be…*in love with me.*

As I burned off the UV Blue in the pool, I replayed moments from the previous night in my head, lap after lap. Images of Chad's jet-black curls and the tightness of his grip helped the workout fly by, but it took every bit of self-control not to smile when he took his place at the lifeguard stand halfway through practice.

We exchanged a coy head nod as I dripped past him on my way to the locker room. Our eyes read, "I see you, I still want to sleep with you, but I respect you as a friend and a person."

I was the last swimmer out of the locker room that morning, taking my time to wash away the remnants of the week. Hell, the whole junior year. It felt right to train with the team again, but only by familiarity. At least practice gave me some structure, a third place that wasn't partying and of course, a workout. Though my recent male interest redirected attention away from my athletic career and its concerns, it misconstrued a core issue: my lack of self-worth. In the shower, I dropped my Speedo near the drain and watched the water roll off my breasts. After workouts, blackouts, hook-ups and a perpetual restriction of caloric intake, this body had borne so much.

"*Skip lunch.*" Said my old friend, Ed.

"*Then he'll really want you.*"

The next 24 hours flew by, and I found myself at my neighbor's house party with Chad. I could tell right away that something in him had shifted, and it wasn't the alcohol. The way he looked at me went from like to lust, and while I had never seen Chad with another woman, talk about another woman, or flirt with another woman, he was certainly pursuing me. Before the two of us got too handsy in front of our peers, we snuck out together and made our way towards my place, which was conveniently two doors down. Where on Thursday, Chad's conscience spoke through each kiss, this night, he dropped any hesitation he might have felt due to Evan.

Evan.

Damnit, Evan. What were the chances Evan wouldn't find out about this love affair? What were the chances Evan would suddenly transfer in his last year at university? What were the chances Evan wouldn't care that I had slept with his best friend, only a week after our own rendezvous?

The answer to all the above was zero. Nope. Absolutely not. Pure, indisputable, rage and resentment would be the only logical response from Evan. Rightfully so, and for good reason.

Evan of course did find out, but for a moment - at least a month - Chad and I didn't care about the repercussions our affair would have on Evan as much as we longed for that tingling between our legs. In fact, Chad and I kept this momentum high, carving time into our schedules so we could be together - or better put, bang. Chad reiterated how happy he was to be with me, and that his friendship with Evan wasn't something to worry about. So, I didn't, because I was happy to be with Chad, too.

There was no pivotal moment when I "found out" that Evan "found out" about me and Chad. We lived on a small campus where shit spreads fast. I tried validating my actions by reminding myself that Evan and I weren't together, that I was an independent, single woman. Chad illustrated a bad boy fantasy for me, and I wanted to hold onto what I could before this dream blew up in smoke. Chad represented the Anti-Evan of rebellion and sexual rejuvenation, where I inhabited the archetype of good-girl-gone-bad.

Come Halloween, the holiday for all hell to break loose, I slipped into my impossibly small, sparkling pink leotard for my debut as Alana "Honey Boo-Boo" Thompson. It was an outlandish and expedient costume, as it reflected the childish behavior I portrayed throughout that fall semester. I acknowledged my trashy antics by diving deep into them, armoring my self-esteem in ironic costume. Though instead of owning up to my actions, I abrasively mocked them.

With a bottle of GoGo Juice in hand, my teammates and I stepped into a sweaty house party at 8pm on a Saturday night. Drunk, I tipped-toed behind my friends with my tutu tight and curls coming loose. The hot pink lipstick I rubbed generously around my lips now covered the rim of my Solo cup. And whatever I'd been drinking from the punch bowl wasn't staying down. I anxiously texted Chad, who I had slept with two nights prior, but hadn't heard from since. My swim friends were ready to leave the party right away, as all our NARP friends were liquored past the point of mingling.

I stood at a crossroads of partying decisions when Evan swept past me only to point and laugh at my get up. Easy for him to mock, as he wasn't in costume. When we dated, he told me that dressing up for Halloween was juvenile as he "didn't see the point of trying to be someone you're not." Which is, at least how I see it, entirely the point.

I grabbed a shot of some stranger's tequila in the kitchen and immediately threw it back up in my cup, dropped it on the counter and skidded away. I figured the hosts would discover worse things at the party and bounced to Chad's.

Curtis opened the door with regret.

"Chad can't see you right now," he said.

'Can't see me?!' I thought, standing drunk, alone, and terribly confused. Chad emerged behind Curtis with squinting eyes and shrugged,

"Sorry Jen, not tonight." He shut the door and I headed home, pouting. Ripping off my leotard, I crawled into bed fully naked and utterly ashamed. Rejection reigned over me – from boys to alcohol, I couldn't hold onto anyone or anything.

The next morning, I awoke at a loss. I had lost control of the relationships in my life, no longer secure in my sexuality. I questioned my ability to attract men and how others perceived me. For so long, I had prided myself on being skinny, confident that I was desirable. I fought to remain thin in my skin so men would pursue me. But maybe being cute and small wasn't enough. Maybe I wasn't enough. Maybe there was something I lacked in order to be loved.

After I washed off the residue of the previous night's makeup, I joined my roommates at the cafeteria, determined to eat away all pain. I circled the breakfast buffet, plate after plate, only slowing down between cups of coffee. Once my roommates vacated, I exchanged seats with a table of volleyball players, grabbing a fresh bowl of honey-laced cereal and another helping of cheesy potatoes.

I spent three hours lingering in the cafeteria that Sunday morning, feeding my low self-worth with brunch while procrastinating on homework. Sluggish, I was sure not to trip over lethargic feet during my three-minute walk home. I could not bear the thought of anyone catching a glimpse of me crossing the street; high on fats and sugar, bloated as can be.

I returned to an empty home, affirming once again: I'm single and alone. Checking my phone for the tenth time, I stared down in disappointment at an empty screen. Chad and I were inseparable all of October, yet his cold and indifferent behavior from Halloween was all that I needed to see that our affair was over.

It all happened so suddenly, my spiraling into Evan's arms one week, and his best friend's the next.

"Jesus, Jenny. You slept with your ex's best friend? That's low. Even for you."

A familiar voice rang in my ears. Passion had consumed all logic, suppressing Ed in the back of my head. Emotions of abandonment, rejection, unworthiness, and shame all surfaced at once. A rush of resentment forged in my midsection, aching for attention. The blood in my stomach pulsated, matching the beating in my chest. Guilt flooded through my limbs. I begged for the bloat to go away, and Ed came to answer my call:

"You can get rid of this, Jenny. You can throw it all up."

As though by a string, my body floated from the living room up to my bathroom. I looked at the puppet staring at me in the mirror before the marionette picked up my toothbrush. I collapsed to the floor, sobbing. "Is this what I'm coming to? Bulimia?" I asked Ed.

Ed's voice paused. I quivered.

"You can make it go away." Ed said once again.

I wanted more than anything to make *it* go away. The food. The pain. The drama. My sexual appetite was ruining the reputations of others, but mostly my own. My actual appetite was now out of my control, so I succumbed to a coping method I had put off for so long. I closed my eyes and took a deep breath. I made it go away.

My fingers gripped into the teal blue bathmat beside my knees. I finally did it. Throw up. I'd always considered the act just in case I overate and wouldn't be able to burn off the food from exercise. After years of calculated restriction, I started to fantasize over forbidden foods, drooling over doughnuts, pizza, French fries and more. Really, any time I refrained from caloric meals with friends and teammates, I imagined myself digging into the hot foods alongside them while slowly crunching on kale. I figured it was a matter of time before my first intentional purge. After the flush, I promised myself to beware of making this a habit. To beware of becoming...
bulimic.

Shortly after Halloween and a couple one-word texts from Chad, Margaret informed me that he "thinks I'm really awesome, but not worth the drama with Evan". I interpreted this message as *"not being worth it."*

The week before Thanksgiving, I "turned-up" on a Tuesday night with my friends on the volleyball team, who had just finished their season. Emotionally, so had I. My fabulously tall friends and I wobbled into a popular bowling alley serving five-dollar pitchers. With the help of our 21-year-old classmates, we chugged domestic drafts while flirting with baseball boys and tweeting on Twitter.

At the time, my Twitter handle was @i_luv_u_jenay with a bio reading, "Narcissistic Thoughts and Drunken Exclamations." As that's what all my tweets implied. I found immense joy in conveying my thoughts to my one hundred followers, most often shared between the hours of 9pm and black out drunk. And on this night, I let the booze do the talking and my thumbs go to work.

Around 6am that next Wednesday morning, my alarm yanked me out of unconsciousness. My boots were still on. My varsity jacket was still on. My makeup was wearing off, but the beer wasn't. I raced across campus to get to a practice I was late to, dreading the next few hours to come.

Jumping into a cold pool had cured all my hangovers in the past, but as I dove in, I realized I wasn't hungover; I was still drunk. Every stroke felt heavy as I dragged my arms through each lap. I waited in the gutter to catch my breath and let my teammates pass me. Flip turns were out of the question as last night's beer kept creeping back up. *Not today, Jenny. Not today.*

I couldn't spot my head coach, but I did see my assistant coach Zane near the empty lifeguard stand. The team was about to begin another round of the set, during which I took the opportunity to hop out and head to the locker room. I pathetically told Zane I was feeling ill while dashing towards the women's bathroom, before he could follow me inside.

I beelined home to take a nap and woke up to a text from Ally:

SMS TEXT:

08:05 AM Ally C: Homie did u quit?

Quit? Quit what? I tapped out at practice this morning, but that was the first time in my college swimming career that I pulled the sick card. And *everyone* gets a free sick card! I reread her message and opened Twitter:

1:07AM @i_luv_u_jenay: I'm quitting swimming and transferring. Too da loo mothafuckersssss!!!!

I couldn't help but giggle. *'Too da loo Motherfuckers'? LOL classic, Jenny.*

Welp. There it was. My drunken exclamation based on a narcissistic thought. Despite my crude language and immature tone, I still thought my tweet was funny as, after all, I was quoting *"The Hangover."* However, I didn't consider the repercussions the tweet would have on my athletic status until my head cleared up hours later.

Throughout the day, other Twitter followers asked if I was truly quitting and transferring, prompting me to delete the tweet and reconsider keeping the app altogether. When passing teammates between classes, I'd catch stink eyes across campus lawns, raising concern around my ostracization. Deflecting the stares and whispers, I wondered if my drunken memos were foreshadowing an expiring swimming career. I didn't expect myself to jump ship, though I fancied the idea of escaping from the hole I kept digging for myself. The weigh-ins, counselors, boy drama, and binging became more suffocating than the waters I dreaded swimming in.

That afternoon I tried to sneak into practice, laying low as I entered the pool deck. "Jenny! Turn around! If you don't want to be on this team, then I don't want you on this team!" My head coach yelled. He pointed towards the exit sign; my expulsion wasn't up for debate. I had royally fucked up. I had disrespected him and my team in under 120 characters on a public forum. As I felt my swimming career slipping out from underneath me, I had to decide whether I wanted to fight to stay on the team.

Again, I had to ask myself: who was I if I wasn't an athlete? Swimming had been my life, my identity. From ages 8 to 18, I was the reigning country club league champion for every event, undefeated with an inflating ego. But as I swam at the competitive level and traveled across the Midwest, I realized there were girls *far* faster than I, so I tried to compete with myself and my own personal times. My excitement for swimming as a teenager cleared a promising trajectory for my college career, though if I was honest, the only numbers I cared about by orientation were L-B's and calories. I arrived on campus eager to immerse myself in the team and culture of being a student athlete, until insecurities of how I looked and who I attracted got in the way of what I thought I wanted. At this point, the title of a swimmer meant clout on campus, something I cared more about than seeing my name on a scoreboard. As a swimmer, I yearned for status, exclusivity, and Nike swag. And my teammates read right through that. Freshman and sophomore year, any other swimmer would say that I was dedicated, but I wasn't eating enough to sustain any power. Though as junior year progressed, my self-care declined. My performance and attitude completely tanked. I was a drag to my coach, my team, and my mental wellbeing, so I set an end goal in sight: make this year on the swim team my last. While I had the option to break my contract with little repercussions, I felt obligated to fulfill the last three months of training. To quit then would only drop another bomb of shame on my psyche.

So, I apologized to my head coach the next day, convinced him I was committed to finishing the season, and started making an exit plan.

...

Come late February, the swim team dialed in to take on our end-of-season conference, but I was checked-out. I continued to drink and smoke leading up to the meet, where I competed in the 400-yard individual medley, the 500-yard freestyle, and for my final race - the mile.

56

On the last day I would ever slip into a $350 FastSkin suit, I slumped behind the blocks, dreading the last 64 laps of my college career. I had dragged in last during my previous two events, well behind the other girls in my heat. There was no doubt I was due for another ass-kicking.

"SWIMMERS TAKE YOUR MARK"

BEEP

"*This is the last 20 minutes of your life as a swimmer!*" I repeated to myself in motivation to stay afloat. I was torn between giving my all and giving up. Swimming had been my pride and joy for all my life, but there was nothing to be proud of when I glided into the wall to cap off this final finish.

I didn't care to check my time. I didn't care to warm down. Instead, I beelined to the showers, let the hot water stream down my back, and shot an airplane bottle of Absolut Vodka. And then another. And then Ally joined me for a third shot before our parents snuck us out of the pool and into a nearby bar for an ice-cold beer.

Neither Ally nor I were twenty-one, but my mom and her dad bought us a draft to commemorate the end of our season. My mom - my biggest cheerleader who had driven across states for years to watch her baby girl do what she loved best, was now supporting my decision to resign. While she recorded every time of every race for *years*, she never once scolded me for a poor performance. She was a swim mom, but she wasn't *that* swim mom. And though we both mourned the end of my career that day, she never alluded to any lost potential. Instead, she bought me a beer, which was the most badass thing I had ever seen her do.

"Wow, Jenny. Look how far you've come... it must be bitter-sweet" my mom consoled on the drive back to the meet.

"Yea, it's... not how I expected I would feel. I thought I would feel more relieved or accomplished. And I know so many swimmers quit before graduation and most quit within a year. I knew it would be hard, but I didn't think it would be *this hard."*

"Yes. But you still tried, and you followed through for three years," she said.

"Yea." I sighed.

I suddenly felt ok disassociating myself from my title, as my identity shifted from "Jenny the swimmer" to "Jenny the *swammer."* I realized that I could be "Jenny-comma-*anything."* And if I wanted to shift my narrative of who I wanted to be, I'd pick another interest and just keep trying.

Back at the pool, Ally and I weaseled our way into the meet without any questions from our team, and I popped a pot brownie in my mouth before the final event: the men's 400 freestyle relay. Thirty-two lengthy, young adults in Speedos huddled behind blocks, jumping up and down to warm up for one last event. From the middle lane, four of my broad-bodied teammates created monstrous waves in the water, fighting their way into first place. The rest of our team shook the bleachers, jumping in celebration for the last big 'W' of the season. By the time the relay team dripped their way up the awards podium, I wasn't just high, I was elated. The weight of responsibility was lifted. No more 5am alarms and forced camaraderie. High and heady, I stepped my toes into Evan's shoes, remembering how isolated he felt being on a team he no longer identified with.

After the meet, our four-hour bus drive back to Cincinnati dragged on as my weed brownie wore off. I could not tell if I overheard my captains Kayla and Heather talking about me, or if it was the paranoia from the pot. Whatever the case, I knew I was only one night away from ever dealing with these bitches again.

Once our bus stopped on campus, fifty swimmers pushed their way out of the retracting door to run home and report back to *the conference party.*

Within the hour of returning from the annual conference meet, it is tradition for the swim team to pop bottles and celebrate the end of a season.

Around 12am, the keg was tapped, and the Jell-O shots were served. By 1am, the team was plastered. The promise of off-season had arrived, keeping the energy level high.

In the middle of a Justin Bieber banger, Caleb, a senior team captain, stormed into the living room and turned off the music. The song stopped mid-chorus of "Boyfriend." *How rude.* Caleb took his hand off the DJ controller and pulled out cash from his back pocket. He turned towards me, waving a twenty-dollar bill.

"This is your refund for the conference party. You know the rules." Caleb lifted the money closer to my face as a wide grin spread across his.

I'm sorry, what?

"Jenny. You broke dry season. Here is your refund. Now go." Like a Boy Scout who ignited his first fire, Caleb could not hide his excitement.

I stood still in shock, tipsy and confused.

Ally stepped in. Her messy bun bounced on the crown of her head as she shouted:

"Back off, Caleb! Every goddamn person on this team has broken dry season! Jenny of all people deserves to stay at this party. And it doesn't matter anyway, she quit!"

O sheeeeeet no one was supposed to know that yet.

Caleb stepped back in shock while my roommates pulled me into the kitchen.

"Don't listen to that loser! He's just butt hurt his swimming career is over and is directing that anger at you." Carly and Lilly comforted me as I considered whether this conundrum was worth resolving. I cultivated disdain from my teammates, after a season of disrespect. I showed up to practices hungover, drunk, and sometimes high, apathetic of competitions and unconcerned about the effects my temperament had on the other swimmers. I could see why my teammates wanted me to leave. And I would, just on my own accord.

The whole Caleb scene really killed my buzz. Slightly more sober, I realized that everyone's suspicion of my resignation was confirmed. Jenny Martin had quit.

Leaving any organization, club or community is almost always bittersweet or despicably bitter. The discrepancy on our team was that a guy could leave and still socialize. But when a woman quit, she was scolded.

For example: Across the beer pong table at the swimmer house, male athletes had etched in ink a list called the "QUITTERS" wall. The names were always female, as the list did not apply to men. Without hesitation, my eyes snapped to a familiar name.

"JENNY"

Not only did my name read thicker and larger than the others, it contained cliff notes:

"THANK GOD"

"FINALLY"

"REHAB?"

Before I could start crying, a former male teammate ushered me upstairs to the attic, where he lived among his ex-teammates. We ripped a bong in his bedroom, talking trash on swimming and how liberating life was without it. No longer was he pretending to conform to feel like he belonged. He had stepped out of the swimmer bubble and onto solid ground.

After a couple bong rips, I checked my phone for the time.

4:37 AM. *Shit!* I had a bus back to Kansas City to catch. I had a spring break to enjoy. It was time for me to leave and go anywhere but *here*.

Eataly

While my infamous "totaloo mutherfuckers" tweet provoked likes, its hubris raised the question: "is this *really* what you want, Jen?" With the short answer being "no," I drew out a long-winded solution to evade my situation all together. I couldn't just quit swimming and transfer, I had to go out in grandiose fashion to prevent the risk of being forgotten. I sought to erase myself from this tumultuous tableau and reframe the narrative of who I was and why I held any significance. Upon stoned brainstorming around my escape plan, the idea dawned on me: flee the country.

After a few meetings with my guidance counselor, I crafted a full report to my parents on why studying abroad would benefit my unclaimed career path. I outlined tuition comparisons and statistics on how such acquired skills could enhance my resume. "What's in this for you?" I presumed in my pitch: "none other than the opportunity to travel when you visit me abroad."

White noise transmitted across the cell phone signal. Eager to elaborate, I let the silence linger as after all, Dad was the one who taught me that when you're selling something, let *them* do most of the talking.

"I'm not going to finance your five-month vacation, Jenny," he said rigidly. "But you've raised some good points." *Finally*, all my thesis papers were being put to effective use. My dad continued; "I suppose travel will teach you to figure things out on your own. But before I say yes to anything, I need to know that you are taking care of yourself."

When we hung up, I flipped open my laptop and hunted down babysitting gigs on a sitter site. It was time I'd stop partying so damn much and show my parents that I was serious about saving for this international stay. During another lengthy phone call, my dad and I reviewed the responsibilities, risks, and privileges it takes to spend five months in another country. In the end, we agreed that this move would inevitably instill some character in me, and my dad signed off for more than one check or document. There were *so many documents*. Especially compared to when I slid into undergrad with a swimming scholarship. No more special treatment, resources, or swag as an athlete. I'd be just another American girl frolicking around Europe.

Originally, I had my heart set on Barcelona. I had studied artists like Antoni Gaudi and Pablo Picasso in high school, romanticizing the idea of how I'd feel strolling along the seaside city. But as I weighed my options and remaining class credits, I found a loophole in my major. If I switched to Public Relations, I could take two required classes in Florence, Italy, and graduate *faster*. And so, I picked Italy, enrolling in an affiliate program which paired me with an apartment full of other American students. Two of my roommates would arrive together from a college in New York while the other two rode solo like me. Minutes after my program emailed over the room assignments, Kylie, one of the girls from New York, had found me on Facebook.

> KYLIE: Hey Jenny! Looks like we'll be living together in Florence! You're super pretty and I'm so excited for us to be friends <3

Omg! I have a friend! Who thinks I'm pretty. Thanks, Kylie, you seem super awesome.

> JENNY: Awe, thanks Kylie! I'm excited too.

> KYLIE: So, the house rules go as follows: Don't get taken, don't get pregnant, and don't get fat. Capisce?

Capisce. Don't get fat. Heard loud and clear, Kylie. Loud and clear.

Anticipating the move to a country known for its food, I exercised vigorously while juggling four part-time gigs to save up for this "trip of a lifetime." It was the summer of 2013, and I had just turned twenty-one. I survived a dozen fake IDs, three years of collegiate swimming, anorexic interventions and had not purged since the previous Halloween. And let us not forget inflicting public humiliation from my drunken decisions and enduring ridicule from others. After evaluating such trials, I was confident I could manage anything, eating disorders and all.

I really was eating more. I was worrying less. I was gaining insight, for sure. But I was still naive to think that studying abroad would flip a switch, opening the door to an infinitely bright future. While my positive disposition allowed me to shine light on dull moments, I suppressed dark tendencies from the entities that burrowed inside my bones. I could not see below the surface, nor was I willing to dig deep.

Despite distracting myself with multiple jobs to prepare for this "trip of a lifetime," no amount of money or air miles could alleviate the thoughts still lingering in my head around food and body image. Ed was not as abrasive this summer, but he still shot me intrusive comments around what I ate and the size of my stomach. He mostly simmered quietly on the backburner until we crossed borders into international cuisines.

The night before my transatlantic flight, I laid awake restless. In fact, the entire week leading up to my semester abroad, a buzz vibrated through me, a foreign feeling from any other drug I had tried before. The transformation had begun. Soon, I'd be crossing cobblestone streets for a frothy cappuccino from a local cafe, where I'd journal each morning before class. In my time of deep reflection in the Renaissance City, I'd transcend into a sophisticated dilettante of high society. I'd return home *golden*.

A toothy smile stretched across my face as I entered security at the Kansas City airport, looking back to wave at my mother, whose cheeks glistened with tears. Three flights separated me from familiarity to foreign land where I was free to explore. Locking eyes with my mom, tears streamed down my cheek, too. This was the last time my mom would see the *old Jenny*.

First stop: a layover in Frankfurt, Germany. *European Territory!* With hours to spare, I strolled through the terminal, gawking at pretzels, strudels, and bier gartens galore. If Europeans were notoriously skinny, why was their food so big? So tempting? So boisterously beautiful? From a kiosk, I bought something baked and brown and headed to my gate.

I overheard a group of young women speaking English and popped over to ask if they were studying abroad.

They were.

In Italy?

They were.

All of you? In Florence, by chance?

Yes, in fact, they were.

I was shocked that this group of twelve or so friends decided to all study abroad together. Wouldn't that defeat the point of immersion and self-exploration? Yet, the group seemed just as surprised to see me traveling alone.

"Aren't you scared? To come here by yourself?" One student asked.

Scared? Scared of what? I was ecstatic. Aroused. Ready. Already in love with this decision and anything but scared.

Boarding my flight to Florence, I stepped into an older, smaller plane that smelt like worn leather. Two girls ripped straight from a Ralph Lauren catalog settled softly in their seats next to me. Whereas I, panting, was the golden retriever in this American Dream.

"Have you been to Europe before?" I yipped.

"Yes," they said without further explanation.

I decided to not bother my seatmates as they scrolled through their phones and gossiped about boys back home. Instead, I gazed dreamily out from my window seat, awaiting our descent. As we dropped, the plane hit turbulence and passengers started to panic. But to me, turbulence signified that the landing was soon approaching. As we pierced through the clouds, a landscape of red rooftops appeared out of thin air. *It's happening!*

I glided through customs, bemused by how easily I passed though the lines. I expected a long ordeal of questioning, but instead I was greeted by a woman with thick black hair that hung by her elbows, framing the sign in her hands that read, "International Student Association." Spotting me and my pink pants from yards away – excuse me, meters away – this woman recognized me as an American student and cheered.

"Ciao! Benvenuta in Italia. I am Lucia, your program director" She grinned through bold, ruby lips. I could have kissed her, but I wasn't sure what was custom quite yet, so I hugged her tightly instead.

"Ciao!" I said. *And so it begins...*

Lucia showed me to the passenger area, where a dozen kids had plopped down on the airport floor with single-serve bottles of prosecco in hand, waiting for the other students to land. I bought my own bottle, clinked with the others, and rejoiced. I had arrived.

As I shook out the last few drops of bubbly onto my tongue, I noticed a familiar face walking through the gate. It was Kylie, strutting in her platinum strands and tanned skin, wearing a black spaghetti-strap top and light washed jeans. Anticipating this greeting, I stood up to meet my new friend in Florence.

"Kylie! Hey roomie! Welcome home." I waved towards her, wagging my pigtail.

Kylie simply smiled, looking just past me, setting her luggage down to pat back her long, blonde hair.

"Mel, is there any Wi-Fi here?" Kylie asked the petite girl beside her.

"Oh... no, I haven't checked." The girl rolled off an annoyed look and turned to me.

"Hey, I'm Mel. You must be Jenny" Mel said softly.

"Yes, Hi Mel! It's so nice to meet you. I can't believe we're here!" I said.

Mel and Kylie looked at me with sealed smiles. Our enthusiasm was not mutual, so I took it they were wiped from flying. Where I, on the other hand, was buzzing from prosecco and infinite possibilities.

Lucia called my name out with a dozen others, assigning shuttles into town. As our van pulled up alongside the airport, I snagged the shotgun seat to gawk out the window, watching architecture age as we inched from the airport into the heart of the city. The buildings developed in character as we weaved through the veins of Florence, with every ornate entranceway towering over its people walking by and through. Wide, wooden doors stood proudly between archways of thick, stone slabs. Larger structures radiated with the power and wealth of the Renaissance, demonstrating sheer imagination and adequate resources the Florentine designers used to create intricate detail and perfect symmetry.

On a smaller scale, residential structures painted in mustard yellow contrasted handsomely against their royal, Roman neighbors. Radio boxes and muffled rants echoed out of windows bordered by evergreen panels, adding another layer of dimension to this sensual symphony.

Up on a wide street corner, a young couple dined under a beige awning labeled "TRATTORIA" in bold, burgundy font. Ivy draped around the storefront, framing the handsome pair. They nearly sat on top of each other, with their faces just a nose length apart. They were in love, and so was I.

Our bus driver pulled the brakes. "*Click.*" As the doors unlocked, I swung mine open and took my first steps in Florence. *"This can't be real."* I thought as my gaze sailed up the side of an ancient apartment that was now new to me.

My four roommates and I lucked out with a city center flat on the first floor of our building. With our luggage in hand, Kylie took the initiative to enter the stone building and head up the stairs. "We're on the first floor." I pointed out.

Kylie thrusted her suitcase up one more step and sighed, "*You* are on the ground floor. *We* are on the first floor." She proceeded by fidgeting with the keys.

"WOMP." We all felt the locks shift. Kylie tried turning the golden, round doorknob to realize it was stagnant and turned the keys one more time. "WOMP." She pushed on the knob and slowly swung our wooden door wide open. One by one, we stepped through in awe, speechless.

The walls of our apartment consisted of walnut oak, covered in classical art. The French doors facing the street casted light onto the oil paintings and detailed furniture. Kylie and Mel migrated to the back, choosing a bedroom for two with ample closet space and no natural light. In the adjacent room, the sunset peered through thick wooden blinds, outlining three beds to choose from between my other roommates, Kate and Jean. On one wall, two twin beds pushed into one, looking limp with nude sheets and a pillow each. The third bed sat across from the other two, between a grand wardrobe and the windows.

Jean slid past me and claimed the single bed, leaving me and Kate to cuddle up for the next five months. We all dropped our luggage to sprawl across our beds.

"I can't believe we're here!" said Kate. Her excitement circuited from her mattress to mine. Kate's thin lips reached towards her ears, further defining the sharp features of her tan face as she beamed.

I looked at Kate, watching her black hair bounce as she danced about in her bed.

"We're really doing this." I sighed.

"Yea." Kate's expression softened into bliss.

A loud yawn came from the opposite side of the room.

"Woo! I'm wiped." Jean said as she started taking off her shoes.

"I'm taking a nap," Jean added.

It occurred to me that I was running off little sleep from the past two days. By now, I was sustaining off pure adrenaline and airline food.

"Same." Kate chimed in. "I'm going to unpack and chill for the night."

I reset with a deep breath and exclaimed: "I'm just getting started."

As Jean and Kate settled in, I asked Kylie and Mel if I could join them for dinner. The three of us blondes immediately caught attention from our male neighbors as we stepped out of our apartment, ignoring the "ciao, bella!" remarks and alluring stares. Mel let out a nervous laugh and Kylie just kept striding forward. I giggled with Mel, feeling like we had just walked into a movie set. The city looked unreal, and the cat calls were right on cue.

Mel and I followed Kylie up to Piazza Signoria, a historic city square of statues and sculptures lining the Palazzo Vecchio, meaning "old palace." Both an archeological site and museum today, the Palazzo Vecchio was one of the first government buildings of Florence, founded in 1299. The old palace resembled a medieval fortress and reminded me of the castles from my childhood picture books. Speared a little off center from the roof of this castle, a clock tower built for Rapunzel struck me that this was about to be a pivotal time in my life. Clueless as to what I was in for, something told me that I was safe to stay.

My eye traced down the golden brick walls of the Palazzo Vecchio to ground level, where half a dozen marble statues stood under gothic vaulted ceilings. We had walked into an outdoor museum of sorts, as I recognized Michaelangelo's Statue of David proudly guarding the doorway entrance.

"That's not actually the Statue of David," Kylie stated.

"I know. It's in the Accademia" I said while admiring its smaller replica.

Kylie remained silent and trailed forward. I kept staring at the erected emblems, bewildered by the art and the Italians' ability to preserve so much of it.

"Jenny!" Kylie called out as a sea of passing tourists started to swallow me into their group.

"We have five months to look around. Let's eat." Kylie led us through a narrow street free of cars and little foot traffic.

"Here, this place looks good. You can tell because the menu is in Italian and there are no cheesy photos." Kylie said as she scanned the framed menu alongside the front door of the trattoria.

"I mean honestly, as long as you avoid restaurants off a main square, you're good. Otherwise, you will pay for overpriced, mediocre food and get hassled by gypsies." she added.

When Kylie was sixteen, she visited her older sister studying abroad in Florence, and thus, I soon learned, knew everything there was to know about Italy.

"Oh, and beware of the fluffy gelato. Again, overrated and overpriced. The best kind is packed down rather than blown up for show."

At our quaint and quiet dinner spot, my roommates ordered tagliatelle Bolognese while I pointed to an item on the menu that read "insalata." When two steaming balls of yellow pasta doused in meat sauce laid down on the table, we all cooed. Our waiter then dropped off my cold plate of pale romaine and shredded seafood. Kylie and Mel shot a confused look at me, and I hastened to explain.

"Mmm... your pasta smells so good. I shouldn't have eaten so much in Frankfurt." I lied in defense.

Come September, "I had a big breakfast" became more ingrained in my vocabulary than anything I learned in my Italian 101 class. My pledge to Kylie to "not get fat" haunted me each time I was invited out to eat. So, I allocated one cheat meal a week and stuck to my grocery list of yogurt, fruit, and salad for the remaining days.

Over the first few months in Florence, I consumed my calories between the hours of 9pm and 3am, as I easily drank a bottle of wine each night I went out, which was all but one night of the week. During a late-night meal, I discovered a love for the greasy, dense, halal kebab. This delightful wrap is crafted from lamb meat (or maybe chicken?) which rotates on a stick beneath a heat lamp all day, then shaved into a flour tortilla topped with lettuce, French fries, tomatoes, tzatziki or hot sauce. For me- tzatziki *and* hot sauce. My first bite into a kebab changed my outlook on life—not in a spiritual way, but in a *you've been starving yourself* kind of way, activating my taste buds to a new level. Kebabs, along with pizza, pasta and gelato completely transformed my tongue as I progressively packed in more sodium meal after meal. I told myself that these salty snacks were liberating me from an anorexic past, that these midnight feasts were acceptable as my only meal for the day. Because once 5pm would come around, I'd uncork the vino rosso I bought for three euros, topping off my glass until the bottle was finished. By the final pour, my inhibitions would lower, evoking me to eat. I didn't care about the calories in margherita pizza so long as wine coursed through my veins. Though by the morning, my head would rumble and my belly would bloat. I'd hit snooze on my alarm and start the countdown for 5pm, when I'd pop another bottle and evade accountability for my body.

I combated initial weight gain with hours of cardio and eating little to no food unless it was accompanied by booze. I joined a gym targeted to international students and ran myself lost around the city, figuring that the longer I was out wandering, the more calories I would burn.

On one of those first runs in August, I ventured over to the south "OltrArno" side of Florence. Meaning 'beyond the Arno River,' this quarter is much quieter than its northern neighbors, where locals mingle to wine and dine.

I started my run on a residential road, trotting through cobblestone lined in the town's ubiquitous beige buildings with green window shades. Following the sunlight, I headed towards a main passage, where I spun out into a crowd of various tour groups. The music from my phone continued to play, but I stopped dead in my tracks to absorb the diversity around me. Korean, Chinese, German and Dutch guides waved batons and umbrellas to signal their designated travelers. Hundreds of humans funneled in and out of the bridge that extended from the road. From a side view, an assortment of tan storefronts stacked up like dominoes along the bridge's archway, with windows, those green window shades, and terracotta awnings suspended along the rooftops. This bridge stuck out considerably from its other boring bridge buddies along the Arno River, which were merely for auto transportation. *Yawn.*

After snoozing off too several European history classes back in Ohio, I conducted a little research before embarking to Italy. The Ponte Vecchio, or "Old Bridge," has been standing since the 14th century. Google taught me that this bridge was once a marketplace for butchers, until the meat reeked so bad that the city council revamped the arch's reputation and started selling gold, jewelry, and other fine goods. One fun fact I found on the interweb was that the Ponte Vecchio was the only bridge that survived German bombs during World War II. Rumor has it that a Nazi official was dating an Italian chick, of whom pleaded with her sweetheart to spare the significant site. *Make love not war, am I right?*

Beneath the bridge lies secret passageways linking the Ponte Vecchio between noble palaces like the Palazzo Vecchio near my apartment. These corridors were commissioned by the Medici family, who basically ruled all of Florence due to their political and fiscal power during the 15th century. I learned this last fact during Lucia's walking tour, which is why I only half-ass my history research before visiting a city, leaving room for surprise.

And to my surprise, the Google Photo I saved as my home screen all summer was now live in 3D. Was I manifesting? Treading lightly, I entered the image that I had glanced at for months, downloading a wave of sensory overload.

The aroma of roasted chestnuts mitigated sewage rank from the river. Children scrambled about, laughing and crying. Tourists moseyed around, haggling and buying. People of all ages and nations wore leather boots, white sneakers, and high heels (*why the high heels?*). Artists painted with oils, gold glittered in the sunlight, and diamonds dazzled behind glass displays. Couples walked slowly, utterly in love. I lovingly walked past them, soaking up the energy of it all.

From Ponte Vecchio, I followed a main road until it split into a fork in four directions. I certainly was not in my suburban hometown of perfect grids and three-lane streets. Along for adventure, I chose *up*. After countless switchbacks shaded by cypress trees, I stopped at a large stone staircase swarming with tourists. Anticipation swelled as I followed the fever radiating off the other foreigners. A plateau of cement cleared across the horizon, where tourists wandered around another replica of the Statue of David. Staring at the iconic centerpiece, I was trying to decipher where I was based on context clues. And then, I turned around.

Bursting with endorphins, I shivered on top of the Piazzale Michelangelo, a world-class site that offers a majestic panorama view of Florence. Scanning a field of terracotta rooftops, I located my apartment by the Piazza Signoria from where I stood, spotting the clock tower emerging from the Palazzo Vecchio. What seemed like a block away, I noticed the Duomo, or the Florence Cathedral, regal in its white, green, and red marble walls. The Duomo, creatively named for its dome-like structure, emerged saliently among the other buildings. I had passed the Duomo before on foot, though this new perspective on top of the hill revealed how truly vast this church is to scale.

I trembled. Was this my white-light spiritual awakening? Or was I just high from the run? Staring down at the renaissance city from the Piazzale Michelangelo, I stepped into a time warp. Everything stopped. My heart rate slowed down. My skin glistened under the Tuscan sun. I listened within as my soul spoke Italian. *Va Bene.*

...

Kikuya is an English pub located in the heart of Florence, a block behind my Italian apartment. This spot notoriously serves the Wells Dragoon Pale Ale, which is a 10% ABV beer guaranteed to get you 100% wasted. This Western bar welcomed international students with affordable drinks and darkly lit rooms. Three weeks into our stay, a half dozen girls from my program huddled in a booth with a Dragoon in each hand. Cher, a student from California, then introduced her take on the drinking game "Thumper." In Thumper, the group begins clapping between their hands and the table to initiate a rhythm. The lead calls out "what are we playing?" in which the group responds, "THUMPER!" The lead asks, "why are we playing?" and receives a response: "TO GET FUCKED UP!" Then, each participant goes around in the circle to announce their signal. The game then begins as players string along signals at random. As the made-up rules state, you cannot choose the gesture that was used right before you, and you can't fuck up the beat. And when you do, you drink.

In Cher's version, we dropped the charades and picked an adjective for "Fuck." For example, we all choose names such as "sexy fuck," "hard fuck," "loud fuck" and so on. When it was Cher's turn to go, she picked "kinky fuck."

Damnit. That was mine!

I didn't have time to improvise, so I picked "freaky fuck". Not as fun as kinky, but close.

As the game started, "sexy fuck" chose "loud fuck," "loud fuck" chose "kinky fuck." Cher opened her mouth for ki…

"I'M KINKY FUCK!" I shouted.

I leaned into Cher, yelling at her for taking my *fucking* adjective. With horror scanned across her face, Cher sunk into her leather seat while I towered over her. The booth of girls went silent. The alcohol took over me. Whatever social conduct I still possessed was slayed by the Dragoon. Gasping, I snapped out of the trance and slowly sat down. I was horrified, unsure how Cher and the rest were about to respond to my recent outburst.

Everyone froze. Then without hesitation, our entire corner of Kikuya burst out into laughter.

"JENNY! What the actual fuck." Cried out Cher.

I whimpered back: "Oh my god. Cher. I'm so sorry. I don't know what just happened. I don't know why I got so angry. That came out of nowhere... I guess... I'm just... a kinky fuck at heart and got carried away."

The group laughed it off, dubbing this incident as a defining moment for my reputation as the fun party girl with a new nickname: kinky fuck. They found me hilarious, applauding my drunken malarky. I wore this title proudly, relived to have found my people in the corner booth of a dim pub.

I laid in bed the next morning assured that these new friends weren't interested in me because of my past or because I was pretty, but that they enjoyed my company and goofy antics. I've never been afraid to laugh at myself. In fact, I often practice laughing at myself since it's easier than taking life too seriously. If you're going to burst out at anything, burst out in laughter. And if you're going to be a freaky fuck, commit to it.

Someone I found struggling to not take themselves too seriously was my roommate Kylie. While she was the first person to ever "connect" with me in Florence, she made no effort to talk to me. Whenever I initiated conversation, I received a one-worded response. Whenever I *was* at the apartment, which was rare and only to sleep and shower - which was also rare - I would find Kylie scrolling through impossibly thin models on Tumblr. The first time I noticed the emaciated figures from Kylie's laptop, it triggered a memory from one night in college when I sat ashamed after eating a gluttonous meal. Ed came through, imploring me to turn to the internet for thinspiration. I typed "skinny" into my web browser and flipped through photos before peeling my eyes away from the screen. Seeing those images ignited more shame than the act of overeating itself. I closed my laptop that day in disgust, ridden with rue as if I had discovered kiddie porn.

Sliding behind Kylie's screen, I reckoned we didn't talk because we had nothing to talk about. Her initial Facebook message was rooted in appearance, but face-to-face, there was nothing to say. I found out from another student that Kylie had sent a similar message about connecting in Italy because that person was pretty. Albeit flattering, I was affronted that Kylie only wanted to be friends based on my looks. Was I wrong in this thinking? Was I being ungrateful, petty, and self-righteous? Then again, all my friends were beautiful. At least, they were beautiful to me. And at least I didn't source girls off the internet. Maybe, my roommate was curating a dream team of girlies to sit VIP in at Europe's hottest clubs. Or maybe, she was just lonely.

That afternoon instilled a shift within my self-image. I did not want to be defined by my looks. I was more than just "the skinny friend." I wanted assurance that my appeal was due to my essence, over my appearance. I needed to trust that my so-called "friends" and prospective partners were not falling for the halo around my head, but that I had a light to offer.

As far as prospective partners went, the only action I got in Italy was a midnight make-out sesh with a Brazilian model. I met Marco right after deciding that I would no longer be bound by beauty, that I would see myself and others for who we really were! No model named Marco could woo me with a chiseled chin and creamy skin, he would have to make me laugh and make me think. And that's just what Marco did one night after buying me a drink. Funny, how hilariously intelligent someone seems when you're under the influence. He was so funny, in fact, I let him kiss me all the way home until we reached my building, where I politely told Marco that this is where our night would end. And as I dreamt of this model's sleepy, opaque eyes, my roommate Kate woke me up to reality the next morning.

"Jenny, don't you have a trip to Venice today?" She asked.

"Shit! Yes, and the tour bus leaves in ten minutes. There's no way I'll make it to the train station in time." I shrieked as I jumped out of bed to throw on yellow shorts and a chambray tank for my first daytrip in Italy.

Running with abandon sans cell phone service, I'd stop to ask any Italian on the street to confirm my direction: "Santa Maria Novella?" I would point out to the distance, scanning the stranger's eyes for reassurance. "Si" they'd respond, and I continued rushing on. Arriving at the bustling station, I valiantly took matters in my own hands and bought a one-way ticket to Venice. My heart rate slowed while I stared out the window of the fast-speed train. Then reasoning crept in. I did not speak Italian, my phone was useless without Wi-Fi, and once we'd stop in Venezia, I'd be proper lost. But I was determined. I marked my calendar to spend that day in Venice and dammit, I was going to spend that day in Venice!

Stepping off the train, I let curiosity lead the way. I shadowed tourists around infamous canals, the magnificent St. Mark's cathedral, and along storefronts displaying a cornucopia of marzipan candies. Confections molded into miniature shapes of watermelon, bananas, peaches, and cherries spread across cake stands behind the window, whispering for me to walk in. So, I did. I picked up a marzipan molded into the shape of an orange, paid for the treat, and took it to a red velvet booth. I picked up the plush orange candy and sunk my teeth into the airbrushed confection, elated as almond extract melted into my mouth. The sugar coursed through my bloodstream as I took out my iPhone and realized that if I spent another minute alone in this town, I'd be stranded from spending all my money on marzipan. I connected to the cafe's Wi-Fi and saw that one of the guides I meant to tour with had messaged me on Facebook.

BROOKLYN: Hey Jenny! This is Brooklyn from EuroTour. We're sorry you missed us this morning, but if you meet us at Saint Mark's Basilica at 3pm, you can catch a ride with us on our way back to Florence.

Phew. For the next few hours, I wandered through vacant side streets, noticing that there weren't any cars in sight. I later learned that there are no wheels allowed in Venice; people must commute by boat or foot. The residential streets exhibited more vibrance than Florence, as bright hues of pink, green and blue stacked above the canals. I warmly nodded at couples and waved back at children with their families gliding on gondolas, debating if I should hop into one myself. The gondolier held a sign charging 60 euros per ride, which cost as much as my train ticket. *Ugh.* I could have avoided this expense if I had set my alarm over making out with Mr. Model. I took a deep breath and decided to take my Instagram shot elsewhere.

As captivated as I was by the town's charm, I fixated on those dang marzipan candies. My mouth salivated for more sugar. My stomach went numb. There was no one stopping me from indulging in another sweet treat.

Behind glass walls, rows of pastel gelato lined up along the window, enticing me in for a taste. I stepped inside the store decorated in emerald wallpaper, round marble tables and cherry oak booths. Approaching the golden register bordered with gummies and chocolates, I pointed to the pistachio tub and requested, "uno." When the cashier handed me my scoop, I felt like I had won a participation ribbon I paid to receive. Then I whipped out my phone and my tongue for a selfie. *Money shot.*

Finding a seat, I dipped my tiny plastic spoon into the mint green whip and popped a dollop in my mouth. The creamy texture shot out fireworks of pleasure in my brain. Two scoops later, the fireworks started to fade. My tummy throbbed at full capacity, and my head ached from the sugar. As I took a big belly breath, my stomach reached over the band of my pants.

Damnit. I sat conflicted as I continued overeating and overthinking, finishing my cup while contemplating another one.

I checked the time and counted the euros in my purse. With ten minutes to spare, I could squeeze in another scoop before meeting Brooklyn and hunted down another gelateria. Before you could say: *una pallina di gelato alla nocciola, per favore*, I was making out with a frozen Nutella cone on a bench, al fresco. French-kissing my Italian ice cream, the bliss of the first bite quickly turned sour. Still, I forced it down my pipe hole. *How romantic.* Dabbing the remnants away from my lips, I cried out "I'm sorry" in my head while holding my belly in my hands. I then stood up, threw away my napkin and slapped on a smile. Shoving this gluttonous act out of my memory like I did the sugar down my throat, I repented with suppression, striding towards St. Mark's Basilica free of sin.

Brooklyn stuck out from the mob of tourists in her branded blue EuroTour shirt. She recognized me instantly, signaling a cordial connection once our smiles synchronized across Piazza San Marco, or St. Mark's square, where pigeons outnumber people flocking about the basilica's Venetian-Byzantine building. Brooklyn headed towards me as I stopped to study the landmark's grandeur. My eyes wandered across opulent archways, marble columns and tiled facades, all glistening from the reflection of the lagoon, adding an imperial glow to this infamous island.

"You must be Jenny." Brooklyn said as she waved me down from my airy stare. Her straight, dark hair hung by her elbows, with bangs framing her face. She had sparkling brown eyes and as she would say, an "Italian nose." Brooklyn was here on scholarship from Rhode Island, finishing her senior year in Italy while interning with EuroTour. She arrived in Italy two weeks prior to I to take an intensive Italian language course, which she mastered effortlessly through her thick New England accent.

"Jeez, Brooklyn! You're like a local." I said during our bus ride back to Florence.

"I'm still learning how to order coffee. It's ess-presso, not ex-presso. Which, of course, you already know" I ex-pressed to my new friend.

"Va bene, Jenny. You can't expect to inherit an entire culture in just five months. You don't need to figure it all out, but it's better when you try." She said as she patted my shoulder.

"Va bene." I replied with relief.

Va bene.

Alright. Okay. It's all going to be okay.

Already fast friends, Brooklyn adapted seamlessly into the girl groups within my program. There were a couple guys included in that group, too, though the ratio of men to women in my program was 1 to 6, which was a dating pool I did not dare jump into. Besides, I was not in Florence to flirt with American boys. If I were to get my fix, I would seek out pleasure in foreign faces that I knew I'd never see again. By November, my dry spell left me restless, and I hoped to get lucky in a city I had so longed to see, Barcelona.

Bar-the-lo-na. *Barthelona.* Oh, how I can't wait to return to Barcelona. I had booked this trip long before I left for Europe as the famously incomplete Sagrada Familia summoned me to observe its ongoing operation. To join me on this journey, I contacted an old friend named Chloe who had briefly swam on my college team before transferring after freshman year. Chloe was incredibly patient and refreshingly sweet. Where in contrast, one might consider me as having a "loud" personality, Chloe was quite reserved. And while Chloe and I were never that close, her essence emitted a softness I could never forget. Chloe was studying in Seville the semester I was in Florence, so we coordinated a long weekend away to this celebrated Spanish city.

Hopping off the taxi from the airport, I heard my name as I checked in at the hostel.

"Jenny!" I turned around to see Chloe, whose hair had deepened into ebony. She added bangs that were adorable on her round face. I noticed how slim she looked in her chest, waist, and shoulders, whereas I was beginning to blow up in such regions.

"Chloe! You look amazing! It's so good to see you!" I said as I threw my arms around my shorter friend.

"Yea this is wild. Together… in Europe!" Chloe's eyes expanded with possibility.

"Dude. I'm on cloud nine. How are you feeling? You ready to make moves?" I asked with luggage still by my side.

"For sure. I figured we can head to the Sagrada Familia first, then head to a tapas restaurant I found with great reviews." Chloe studied my reaction to her tentative plans. We made a soft itinerary of must-sees while chatting online, but the only activities I was firm on was where we would party. Otherwise, I was more than happy that Chloe would take the lead.

"Hell yea!" I lunged towards Chloe for a squeeze. If we were both dogs, she'd be the one quietly wagging her tail beside me, while I'd be the one jumping and barking when our human came home.

"Sorry… I'm a lot…I'm just so, *so* excited to be here." I backed off, still smiling.

"Jenny… you're the perfect amount of enough."

Walking towards the Sagrada Familia, the cosmopolitan city pulsed with vitality. Barcelona's wide urban streets, glass skyscrapers, and pervasive globalization compared drastically to Florence's well-preserved, homogeneous essence. The red and yellow striped Catalonian flag hung over every street corner, waving a ubiquitous reminder of the city's autonomy and individuality. Once we crossed a couple steep hills from the hostel, Chloe tapped my shoulder and pointed ahead.

"Look!" She whispered.

"Ah!" I screamed.

Through the tops of wide, evergreen oak trees, four pillars shot out from the horizon, with golden spheres glowing from the tip of each one. Two industrial cranes lingered above these hallowed columns looking like erected cheese graters. As Chloe and I inched closer to the UNESCO World Heritage Site, marvel shifted into monstrosity once we approached the line of people crowding the sidewalk.

Thousands of tourists swarmed around the iconic structure. This unfinished masterpiece of ornate sculptures, geometric facades, pinnacles, and pillars continues to build off the blueprints of the late architect Antonio Guadi. The Neo-Gothic elements of the original sketches offer a futuristic design to this highly anticipated project. Commenced in 1883, the Temple is projected to finish in 2026 for the 100th anniversary of Guadi's death, though has since been pushed back due to COVID-19. However, when Chloe and I witnessed the work in progress in 2013, people had no problem packing themselves in and out of the astonishing site.

Chloe and I snuck up as close as possible without paying for a ticket, spending a good half hour around the circumference of the facade. Gothic buttresses supported the entrance in a warped way, creating an optical illusion for a container holding the most powerful wonder of all: God.

"Chloe." I turned to my friend, who looked just as stunned as I.

"When it's finished, we're coming back. We'll stay in a hotel and buy a fast-pass ticket to experience it from the inside." I said, projecting my daydream.

"Oh, I can get on board with that." Chloe confirmed, daydreaming beside me.

"Welp. Now that we aren't spending 60 euros on a four-hour tour, you ready to eat?" I asked, waiting for this moment all day. After snacking on baked goods and crackers in the airport, I was eager to sink my teeth into something hot.

"Yes!" Chloe said. "Follow me."

Chloe led us into a cozy bodega with Rioja red walls covered in black and white photos and vintage posters. We split an order of patatas bravas, Spanish ham, sharp cheese, and a pitcher of apple-infused red sangria. While the food arrived plate after plate, none of which filled me up. The patatas bravas, a popular potato dish smothered in spicy tomato sauce, brought my mouth to salivate in the first bite. But as I continued to push potatoes down my throat, I lost lubrication as my stomach reached capacity. Every physiological sign pointed to "full" as my belly rumbled, and burps let out. And while it pained me to do so, I continued to eat, fetching another savory hit of delicious dopamine.

I noticed Chloe eating at a much slower rate than I, making me inclined to want to eat *more*, in a weird, irritating way. I could hear whispers of Ed echo while Chloe told me about her sweetheart back home.

"She has so much more control than you do. See how she politely picks at her food? And knows when to stop? No wonder she has a boyfriend..." hissed Ed.

I tried shaking off Ed's commentary to focus on Chloe, though my thoughts kept directing me back to the food: The food I had just devoured, the smaller amount of food Chloe had eaten, the food still left on the table, the food being served to the guests around us, and the prospect of more food in the future.

Thinking about all this food, I steered the conversation away from Chloe to bitch about my inclining weight gain.

"The scale keeps creeping up, Chloe!" I threw up my hands for dramatic effect, fishing for validation as "getting fat" was my biggest fear beginning to manifest. We had all weekend to talk about Chloe's partner. I needed reassurance that afternoon before any more imbibing.

"You do and have always looked amazing, Jenny. But you know that's not why I appreciate you. Don't be so hard on yourself." Chloe replied honestly as she finished her first glass of sangria.

I paused to sip the remains of my third pour from the pitcher. She said what I expected to hear, but her sincerity did not heal what I was not willing to accept.

"Well thanks, Chloe. You're right, I shouldn't let a little weight gain get to me... I just want to feel desirable again."

When it came to perceived desirability, drinking played a strong role. Chloe and I ventured off to Opium, a famous beachside club filled with plush white couches, violet ambiance lighting and horny guests from all around the world. Minutes after making it to the dancefloor, I traded Chloe for a tall, lean French man. Together, we ran towards the sea and made out in the sand. We laid under the moonlight, with enough reflection streaming from the sky to spot the rose in our cheeks and light in our eyes.

"You're so beautiful." He said leaning over me. I could have been buried in that moment, dying a drunk, happy girl.

"Merci beaucoup." I said in my best French accent.

He kissed me again as we laid there, then got up to retreat to his friends. Reaching out a hand to help me up, he kissed my knuckles as I rose to stand.

"Be well, you beautiful American woman. It's my best friend's birthday... I must go." He took my hand to his neck to draw me in, kissed me one last time, then ran down the beach to join his entourage. Before returning to the club to find Chloe, I gazed across the black waters on the horizon, replaying the scenes of the day in my head. I wanted to feel desirable, and for a moment, I did. But my desirability stood on precarious conditions of external systems, fleeting like the feeling of the first bite of any dish, or the sweet kiss of an anonymous man.

The next morning, Chloe and I ventured over to Parque Guell, another stunning destination designed by Antonio Guadi. I sported sunglasses the entire time, too hungover to pose without them as we took photos under the Greek Theatre, a regal hallway of thick Doric columns holding up a rooftop of concave mosaics with frosted white and blue tiles. We had stepped into a Dr. Seuss book, or maybe, Atlantis. If such a utopia existed, then surely Guadi was dispatched from the lost city to recreate a version here on earth, in Barcelona.

On top of the fantastical columns lies a balcony overlooking the city's skyline and two plump, cobblestone homes sporting bright, checkered rooftops. These were Guadi's homes turned into gift shops but looked more like Hansel and Gretel's gingerbread house to me. Edging the balcony, I laid back onto a bench of tiled motifs, in which my tired bones molded into perfectly. Chloe and I sat on top of the city in silence, watching people and cars and the time go by. We basked in the Spanish sun, honoring the park's ingenuity with admiration.

Twenty minutes had passed upon that ledge when I heard the rumble in my stomach.

"Yo Chloe... I'm hungry. You mind if we leave to eat?" I implored despite having just shared toasted, sugar-coated churros dipped in thick, melted cocoa.

"Sure, we can head over the Central Market. You can pick out whatever, but I'm good for now." Chloe agreed kindly.

My hunger had me vexed. Why couldn't I match Chloe's eating habits? As each hour passed with my travel buddy, I grew more irritable as an impending binge arrested at the hands of humility. All I wanted was indulgence, but I had to consider my innocent, temperate friend.

...

Las Ramblas is a must-visit pedestrian thoroughfare lined with elm and palm trees, statues, shops, and elegant restaurants. Off Las Ramblas lies the mecca of all markets: La Boqueria. Simulating the frenzy of a festival, La Boqueria attracts crowds in through an entrance awning that's set up like a stage, offering a culinary experience for a wide variety of tastes.

The alluring hype drew Chloe and I into the market to feast our senses on incredible, edible things. Raw meat hung down one side of the hall, with decapitated pig heads watching people from a sheet of ice. A captivating sight, but not what I was in the market for. Chloe and I veered left to a wall of fruit organized into plastic cups stacked ten feet above our heads. Strawberries and mango, papaya and cantaloupe, kiwi, and honeydew. All one euro each. I bought sliced mangos and noticed I was low on the cash I had allotted for the day, then kept my eyes peeled for another cheap treat.

"Ok, I'm ready for a snack. I'm getting a ham cone." Chloe said.

"A ham cone?" I balked.

"Yea, ibérico ham. It's like a delicacy here and it's hard to come by in the states."

"That's ridiculous. Americans are meatheads. Why aren't we importing this stuff like we do wine? Or just... make it ourselves?" I wondered.

"The imports are absurdly expensive. And we don't make it back home because dry cured meat doesn't meet American food standards." Chloe answered.

"Ah, but the dollar quarter pounder passes for quality grade meat. Makes sense." I teased.

"Literally so backwards." Chloe agreed.

"Well hey, let's split for a bit. You grab your meat cone. I'm going to shop for gifts." I suggested.

"Just don't buy any meat." Chloe joked. "It won't get through customs."

Parting ways, I meandered through La Boqueria to find a merchant selling marzipan, displaying dozens of different bright, creative confections. Molded pears, peaches, lemons, limes, and cherries created shelves of "fruit." Near the bottom of the display, sushi rolls, ice cream cones and small packs of McDonald's French fries sat in baskets only an arm's length away.

I picked up tongs and a plastic bag to fill with fondant fruit, affording three pieces while leaving a few more euros to spare. I popped a cherry marzipan in my mouth and welcomed in a rush of activated pleasure receptors. The candy melted immediately, shooting off sweet sensations to my brain. Saving the other two pieces in my purse, I found Chloe and joined her for a 2 euro meat cone.

"You want the rest of mine? I'm full." Chloe offered after her first bite.

Full? What is full? And what does that feel like? After the past three years of restriction, I could tell you how many calories were on my plate, but I could not tell if I was hungry, because I was *always* hungry. I didn't know hunger because I lived in pain. Now, I lived in hunger, and restriction became an obsolete tactic.

My clothes started to tighten in Spain, but I kept eating anyway. After leaving La Boqueria, we strolled through swanky neighborhoods, lush with ivy draping down balconies. Entering a shopping district, we stepped inside a Stradivarius to accommodate my expanding waistline. The changing room's fluorescent lights revealed a disturbing truth as I drew the curtain, revolted by my reflection. My soft stomach started to fold over the size 2 skirt. Unzipping the back of the garment, I let out the breath keeping my belly snatched and cried.

What is happening to me? Where did my 00 body go? Why can't I just go back to the days where I could sustain off apples and string cheese and why, for the love of God, can I not stop eating?

Between meals, all I thought about was more meals. During meals, I told myself, "Fuck it. You'll work out more and eat less tomorrow." Though as I waited in line at the store with a stretchy skirt and a flowy top from the sale section, I gripped onto the price tags with dread, seeing how all the money I was spending on food would cost me a whole new wardrobe. After leaving the register as an indifferent customer, I snapped out of my self-pity and focused on the evening ahead. I would slap on some lipstick, rock this new outfit, and drink away any remorse for my recent weight gain.

Chloe had coordinated plans with her study abroad friends who were also in town from Seville. We bought tickets to Razzmatazz, one of the city's largest nightclubs containing five music halls and an abundance of sweaty, drug-induced dancers. As Chloe and I revisited Las Ramblas, we batted off drug dealers and unsolicited cat calls on the strip as we headed towards her friends. Before entering their hostel, she stopped me.

"I want to make it home at a reasonable hour tonight, Jenny. I've got an early flight tomorrow" she said with hesitation.

"Yea, yea. Sure thing" I shot back.

That's cute, Chloe. Considering it's already 11pm and Razzmatazz opens at one.

While my high school Spanish class inspired my visit to Barcelona, it also provoked cautionary tales of notorious pit pocketers. Thus, I gripped tightly to my belongings every waking minute during this trip in Spain. Though once I stepped foot inside the smoky, lasered rooms of Razzmatazz, my worries evaporated. I awoke around noon the next day and Chloe was nowhere to be found. But what I did find were photos of me smoking a joint with an Australian woman I remember ditching Chloe for upon entering the venue. Faded doesn't even *begin* to describe my state as marijuana surely wasn't the only drug wrapped in the doobie I shared with said Australian woman on the club's rooftop, as documented in my photos. Among my many regrets of the evening, the first one that stuck out was how willingly I gave a stranger my phone to capture myself and another stranger partake in illicit drugs.

"RRRRRRRR.."

My top bunk rattled in the hostel bedroom. What I initially thought was construction noise was unfortunately coming from within the building, below my bed. Chloe complained about the snoring keeping her up the night before, but I was too sedated by sangria to notice.

"RRRRRRRAAAAAAHHHHH."

O shit... Chloe!

I didn't get to say goodbye to the travel buddy I had coerced into clubbing. Riddled in guilt, I apologized for ditching her at Razzmatazz in a Facebook message, wishing her well and thanking her for a good time. I'm not sure if she enjoyed her time with me, considering I spent it scouting for men and complaining about my weight. Yet after she responded with an "it's all good," something else remained trapped inside my blacked-out consciousness. Something shameful. I tried to retrace the memories by looking through photos and messages, but everything remained a blur.

Shortly after my flight back to Italy, I reunited with my Florence friends at Kikuya. We played a couple rounds of Thumper and started sharing travel stories. A friend started talking about her time in Barcelona, visiting the beach, La Boqueria, and her night at Razzmatazz. Then, abruptly, I shouted:

"I HAD SEX AT RAZZMATAZZ!"

A fuzzy image of my body pushed up against a wall with my skirt up to my belly button appeared in my mind, with a blurred man and his skinny wiener thrusting into me. I was having a flashback from the weekend, just then realizing that I had intercourse in public. I had locked eyes and lips with another Frenchman from which I later pieced together was the curly haired dude who dropped me a friend request that Sunday morning. Though it wasn't until the next time I consumed heavy liquor that the gross memory was triggered, making myself and my gal pals all too aware of what I had done during my trip to Barcelona.

Once again, the group sank into silence before a roar of laughter and a melody of "What the fuck?" emerged from those bloody booths at our beloved British bar. I laughed along, only to ease the foul truth around my search for intimacy.

...

Perhaps I was having sex, drunken sex, but I had stopped feeling sexy. By November, I had outgrown most of my clothes, feeling defeated by my lack of willpower. My girlfriends were my redeeming feature, as we had all put on and pound or two and cheered to being "fat, broke and happy." However, I was pushing a 7 kilo add according to the scale at my Italian gym, which is roughly 15 pounds. By the time I returned home to Kansas City, I had gained twenty-two. At the beginning of my stay, I journaled in gratitude and blogged about my weekend excursions, kept focused on my pass-fail classes, and overall felt truly, truly blessed. I was able to travel to eleven countries that semester, seeing bits and pieces of Europe and a fraction of Morocco. My parents, heck my grandparents visited me in Europe, and it is because of them I was able to afford so many excursions. However, the six thousand in savings I earned over the summer shriveled up when I returned from Marrakesh in November, where I splurged on spa treatments that were just so much cheaper than what I would find back home. So like, I couldn't *not* pay ninety dollars for a mud bath and massage at a hammam, where I was steamed, scrubbed, and soaked butt-ass naked in full-ass bliss. And while the camel rides were a must, repelling down the Atlas Mountains was an added excursion I probably could have lived without, yet signed up for anyway. And when I got to the summit of the dusty mountain tops, you know I snapped that money shot to post on Instagram.

By the end of 2013, I was under the spell of Instagram's advent era and had caught the #wanderlust travel bug. My self-image laid in the likes and comments of the few friends that were following me back home. Yet with every pretty photo I posted of a pretty girl in front of a pretty background, my social media stats rose. My taste for adventure exceeded my hunger for likes, yet with this added online attention, I found a new thrill to chase outside the scope of food, booze, and boys.

Where I shared copious photos of famous landmarks and landscapes, I wasn't sharing with anyone how my intrusive thoughts had shifted. Ed's demands deviated from "NO!" and "STOP!" to murmuring lines like, *"You've already lost control. You think you'll go back to a 00? Just buy another slice of pizza, dammit. You don't deserve to be thin."*

At the beginning of the semester, I was eating sporadically, managing my weight with intensive exercise. If I were to pick up a kebab after an Irish Exit from the bars, I compensated with strict restrictions the next day. But by November, a few hours on the elliptical wouldn't burn off the additional 1,000 calories of street food I was consuming late at night.

During those colder days of early winter, I started to shake each morning with anxiety, both from the previous night's booze and my impending graduation date, in which I had no career plans lined up post college. With a month left in my program, I implored my dad to wire me money, since I was dead broke with no credit. This took a tough conversation where my dad outlined the essence of this entitlement, before grudgingly sending over cash. While thankful for the support, dad's advance left me ashamed for mismanaging my money. So, I decided to make some more of it on my own.

At the beginning of the semester, I met a girl who was nannying for an Italian family after class, which inspired me to set up my own profile on sitter sites. For months, I had no bites. Then, with weeks left in my stay, one Italian mom inquired.

Donatella Luis was an English-speaking accountant married to a lawyer, looking for a native English speaker to watch her toddlers after daycare as she wrapped up her workday and prepared dinner. The rate was 40 euros for two hours of help, including dinner. Thrilled to find a nanny with an American dialect, Donatella welcomed me into her suburban home with open arms and gleefully introduced me to Mario, age three and Angelica, age two. I was just as thrilled, as this was an opportunity to immerse myself first-hand inside an Italian home, plus make some extra cash. I had spent so much of my money and time partying that semester, I figured that adding responsibility to my plate would be good for me. And with all the au pairs I had met in Europe, nannying full-time for a foreign family was an option I was starting to consider for a job out of college, and what better option lay ahead than this one to test the waters before diving headfirst?

The kids were cute, they really were. One afternoon in their modern, two-story home, Donatella waved me away from a puzzle with the children to show me a photo album. It was a collection from when Donatella was my age, back when she traveled as a model. As she flipped through scenes of her laying in a bikini off the shores of San Francisco and the French Riviera, she pointed up to her professionally printed maternity photo hanging on the wall.

"That was when I was 35 weeks pregnant with Mario." She beamed.

"You know... I am sixty now." She added.

Sixty years old? With toddlers? I contemplated the biological probability of these two little miracles conceived by a woman Donatella's age. I found it a bit odd she flaunted her modeling photos and pregnancy details so abruptly, though I figured she was just building rapport. And so was I, considering she was the one handing me a meal and money at the end of each visit.

"Hmm..." I looked up at the retired model, with her hair just as full as when she was my age, a mane of sleek black strands with soft waves that ran free down her back. I turned to look across the room at the kids, whose eyes were both as blue and clear as the Mediterranean Sea. I stared back into Donatella's dark eyes and long, thin face.

"Your family is beautiful." I said as Mario started slamming his toys together.

Donatella let out a sigh and nodded towards her kids. "Va bene. Back to the children. I must prepare dinner."

On any given night, Donatella whipped up a simple dish of pasta, poultry, or fresh seafood accompanied with bread, olive oil and red wine. She would stir up plain spaghetti with pomodoro sauce made from plump tomatoes, garlic cloves and basil from her herb garden with ease, orchestrating a melody of ingredients together in such a short amount of time.

"Jenny!" Donatella cried from the kitchen as I was building a fortress of blocks with Mario in the living room.

"What are you doing? It is time to eat. Get the children ready for dinner!" She yelled as if the food would explode if we didn't start dining immediately. Mario looked up at me from his construction of primary-colored plastic, opened a sinister smile and shoved the blocks over into smithereens.

"*Mario...*" I said firmly, careful not to cause any more rise out of this ornery boy.

"Let's clean up your toys and wash our hands." I said to Mario. He resisted and ran towards his mother. Meanwhile, his sister Angelica sat indiscrete, gnawing on a pair of jelly jumbo keys.

"Ugh!" Donatella rolled her eyes as she picked her son up and took him to the bathroom herself to wash his hands. I picked up Angelica and in doing so, startled her. I handed Angelica off to Donatella in front of the bathroom sink, trading her for Mario. Holding Mario on my hip on the way to his highchair, he smiled at me again with those wide deceiving eyes.

"MAMA!" He yelled, his eyes starting to water. He resisted the chair, wiggling around in my arms until mama came out of the bathroom. Donatella sat Angelica in her pink dining seat and turned towards me and Mario.

"Mario, mi bambino." She cooed.

Mario softened the stronghold he had on me, reached out for his mom, and swung from her arms easily into his high seat. I let out a sigh and recalibrated. Once the children sat in their highchairs, the energy of the room felt a little more at peace. I was surely more relieved, as this meant we were about to eat.

Most evenings, my shift ended when the children were fed and their father had returned from work. Mr. Luis had a round face, a bald head, and a cute, wide smile that matched Angelica's. He looked like he could be in his sixties, dressed in silk suits and Gucci loafers, and spoke little English. I looked forward to Mr. Luis's arrival from his job at the law firm, as he symbolized the end of my shift and mitigated any tension in the house. The children were quieter when he was around, and Donatella eased into a better mood. Indubitably, she left me on a high note.

"Grazie mille, Jenny. We are so lucky to have found an American girl like you. The children love you so much. You've been their favorite nanny. See you tomorrow." No matter how annoyed she seemed throughout any given shift, Donatella flattered me when she handed me forty euros cash. My pocket burned as I considered my financial options on the bus ride home. Would I save up for an Italian leather purse? Spend it on a night out with my friends? Or pay back my dad for his recent wire?

"*EAT!*" The voice preceded the urge. Ed was at it again, convincing me that my time in Italy was running up, that I should stuff myself to slow things down.

I jumped off the bus a couple stops before my street, where a glass storefront with the words "PANINERIA" painted on the window caught my eye. I stepped inside the small sandwich shop, where the aroma of rising wheat blossomed up my nose. Behind a glass display, rows of mortadella, pancetta, and melanzane sandwiches stacked up by the cashier. I handed over my crisp new cash for a 4 euro snack of focaccia bread, buffalo mozzarella and thinly sliced prosciutto. The cashier placed my panino into a folded sheet

93

of white paper and handed me my meal and change. Taking my snack outside, I leaned against the side of the building and drooled over my first bite.

I opened my mouth and my stomach rumbled.

"You're not hungry! You JUST ate!" A shot of regret rushed through my consciousness, but my hands did not seem to listen to the signals.

I brought the golden toast up to my lips, tasting the brushed layer of olive oil and salt before my teeth sunk into the pillow of white cheese and marbled meat. Shots fired; I chewed my way into euphoria. Though a few bites later, the high nosedived as my tastebuds resigned. Lethargy passed through me like a wave, and nausea stirred in my core. Part of me wanted to head straight to the gym, part of me wanted to just walk it off. Though most of me was not content, not even in the slightest.

This habit continued each time I commuted back from Donatella's, floating from cafe to cafe as I made my way home. "Food-hopping," as I called it, but only to myself as I never dared to admit this act to my friends, of whom I hoped wouldn't catch me eating in isolation. One afternoon, I ate a Nutella crepe off a popular piazza, spotting Kylie and Mel and their skinny little bodies across the square. Panicked, I picked up my thin pancake in its checkered wrapper and slid into a side street, shoving it in my mouth as I turned my back to my roommates in the distance. With my back against the street, I licked chocolate residue underneath my fingernails, crumpling the wrapper into my pocket. When I looked up, I caught my reflection in a storefront window, revealing brown smudges across my mouth. Inching my head closer to spot check my face, I did not recognize the girl in the glass. We shared similar features, but there was a dullness in her eyes that looked lifeless and afraid.

The more I ate, the more anxious I became. I was losing grip of my concept of control and was falling back into the arms of Ed. As a senior in college, my only objective after this trip was to lose the weight I was rapidly putting on. My younger friends had internships lined up for them back home, while all I had planned was to work up a sweat at my parent's gym.

I had given little thought to what I wanted to do after graduation. However, after months of rampaging through Europe, I knew what I *didn't* want to do. My friends in Kansas and Ohio had committed to salaried jobs with Forbes 500 companies or enrolled into graduate school. The thought of putting myself in their office-appropriate heels made me sicker than my binges. If traveling meant I would risk putting on 10-20 pounds, then I'd take that chance over submitting to the 9-5.

This semester abroad ignited expansion within me, and not just in my pant size. I realized that we are all pretty similar, us humans. We all have families and responsibilities, dreams and drama. We are all working through problems and no matter how pretty or rich or accomplished we are, our shit still stinks. There may be eight billion different hues of skin, but we all bleed red. And whatever blood type we may be, I know one thing: we all need to *breathe.*

The stereotypes I learned from pop culture and my Midwestern upbringing taught me that Italians were loud, well-dressed, well-mannered, and no-nonsense people, unless it came to fútbol. Working for the Luis family near the end of my stay addressed those stereotypes, but who was I to judge?

I had spent most nights in Europe with a blood alcohol level of legally blitzed. I never learned much Italian, though I tried my best to learn my way around the city and the significance of its historical landmarks. This effort of geographical awareness was not so common amongst the other students, unfortunately, as I had some cringing conversations with trust fund babies referring to the Ponte Vecchio bridge as "the pretty one."

Some American students arrived in Italy as a rite of passage, taking pass/fail classes in exchange for university credits, and an excuse to roam freely around Europe with daddy's money. Admittedly, I fell into this mindset, before wanting to fall out. So many of my peers talked of the nepotistic connections they had with powerful agencies in a big city, where they were handed an internship that would lead to a job. Talks about the "real world" prompted me to question the terms of my current reality, seeing that this trip was possible with the financial help of my dad. Though the money was not easily handed to me; my parents and I discussed the value of this allowance, and I did my share of earning my own. After blowing every penny in those short five months, I contemplated all the ways I could persevere in this privileged lifestyle of travel without the subsidy from my parents.

I did not quite know what I wanted to do, but I wanted to keep traveling, to keep challenging the norms of what my peers were up to and what my parents wanted me to do. While I had no plan, I had grit. And that was all it took to figure out the details of my next escape.

...

With a week left in my program, I opened Facebook for a mindless scroll, only to stop dead at the first photo that jumped out at me. A classmate from Ohio had tagged Chad and his impressionable grin in a photo in front of Rome's Colosseum. Curious, I clicked on Chad's profile, noticing he had been bouncing around from Rome to Cannes, and all over Greece. My heart melted. Not for Chad, but for whatever lifestyle enabled all this travel. To inquire, I opened the chat box:

Jenny: Hey I saw Katie Ryan's picture of you in Rome last week. I'm living in Florence – let me know if you get the chance to visit!

Chad: I had no idea. I was just in Florence a couple days ago. I wish I had known. How is it?

Jenny: O bummer! Omg I'm in love. I'm trying to live here after graduation. I never want to leave. So where are you now?

Chad: I'm in Lisbon today and was in Gibraltar yesterday. I agree with wanting to live abroad... No comparison

Jenny: O I'm jealous! I'd love to see Lisbon but I won't make it this time around in Europe. So are you in a different city every day? I want your job.

Chad: Yea pretty much. We were up in the Baltics for a couple months seeing Russia, Germany, Iceland, Norway things like that now were doing the Med. How are things in Florence? That's awesome

Jenny: That's so neat. What's the company you work for? Florence is great. I feel so high on life and I love traveling every weekend. Though I haven't learned much Italian which I feel like I should be

Chad: Haha I just saw your photo from Dublin – I went to the same pub last month. I work for Galleries at Sea so check it out. Don't worry about the Italian. Glad to hear you are having a good time

Jenny: Dublin was great. Everyone was so friendly, spoke English, and were all hammered by noon. I'll have to! I told my parents I won't be living in America after graduation. I'm set on moving around

Chad: hahaha i am 100% w/ you on that one the rest of the world is so friendly

I closed out the chat box and opened Google to search "Galleries at Sea." The polished site was formal, with artworks sliding across the head banner with the title, "Live Auctions Across the Seven Seas." I scrolled through the bottom of the page to the "Careers" tab and applied for an entry position: Art Associate.

The Italian Job

That final semester back in Ohio was one short, foggy phase. As I watched "the best four years of my life" diminish, I held on tightly to the memories from my recent "trip of a lifetime." My college friends and I partied harder and longer when I returned to Cincinnati in January of 2014, upping our antics, and catching the psychosomatic, academic apathy of "senioritis." Though my friends were glad to have their drinking buddy back, they didn't care for the details of Italy and were exhausted by my weight complaints. This sent me into isolation and extreme dieting, often resulting in a binge, and occasionally, a purge. While I shared such behaviors with no one, I clung tightly to the people who were genuinely happy for me, inspired by my adventures and excited to see where I'd end up next. This external validation motivated me to keep moving, and so I kept my head high in the sky, following that clout.

A month after I applied to Galleries at Sea, I interviewed three times over Skype before accepting my position as Art Associate. However, I'd still need to pass a training in Miami before signing onto any assignment across the Seven Seas.

Following the final interview, my parents flew to Cincinnati for a visit but more importantly, to attend a college basketball game. My swim meets had interfered with the basketball schedule in the past, so my dad was relieved to spend the weekend listening to sneakers squeak on the court opposed to sweating on top of galvanized bleachers in a humid natatorium. I was just relieved that my parents came to visit the same week I committed to my "big girl job," and could not wait to share the news.

"Ok! I have a toast to make." I said, raising my red sangria to meet my mom's, hinting at my dad to raise his iced tea. We sat at a trendy Mexican restaurant in downtown Cincinnati, the kind of place where you pay for chips and salsa.

"First off, thank you. For everything. For my tuition and this past semester in Italy." I started.

"You mean your five-month vacation?" My dad said with a strong dose of sarcasm. I lowered my glass to the table, upset by his interruption.

"I'm just joking, Jenny. Your mother and I have seen a significant difference in you since Europe. You've grown more independent, decisive and responsible. But if you want to travel again, it's on your dime. Come May, you're off the payroll." He added.

I took a breath before continuing with my toast.

"That's what I'm getting to. Earlier this week, I accepted a job…on the cruise ships I told you about!" I picked up my sangria and clicked both of my parents' glasses, watching their faces harden into stone. I took a sip, waited for a response, then filled the silence.

"I'll go to Miami in July for training, then who knows… I could go anywhere!" Another sip went down and still, nothing.

"Not only will this job allow me to travel and eat for free, I'll live onboard without any expenses. It's a perfect fit." I waited for a smile to break from either parent, but they looked as dead as the air.

"Dad." I looked right at him, whose eyes stayed locked on the ceiling.

"It's a sales job. I thought that's what you wanted for me." I said.

"I didn't pay for your tuition so you could work on a boat." He grumbled.

"It's a cruise ship, working for a global company." I pleaded.

"How are you paying for your training in Miami? What about May and June? How are you going to make money at the beginning of the summer?" My mom took a jab, ready to fire off another hundred thoughts.

"So, remember that Italian family I babysat for? The mom just emailed me and asked if I would come back and nanny during the interim. She offered to pay for my flights, my food and will put me in a room."

"She's not paying you?" My dad interjected.

"She is. Not a ton, but a weekly stipend of something." I said.

"Why do you need to go to Italy? Why can't you wait tables in Kansas City? Steve Conklin's daughter makes great tips working on the plaza. You'll make more money than what that woman is paying you." He suggested in distress.

I sighed. "Sure, but this is a travel opportunity that fell into my lap. I'm still young, so why not take it?"

"Jenny, you can't just travel. You've got to get a job. A real job. You've got to make money."

Doubts, fears, and frustration fueled the conversation and concluded with how freaking lucky I was to be in my disposition at this time of technology. My parents couldn't and didn't travel like I had at my age. My dad mobilized from the poverty line into a proud owner of nice properties, luxury cars and country club memberships. Through his eyes, I was riding off his coattails, unwilling to do the work to obtain the status of a world traveler. But my parents would not disown me for going against the conventional careers they imagined I'd pursue. Could they blame me, though? With their genes, I was stubborn like my dad and restless like my mom. Choosing adventure over an office was not a bad thing... it just wasn't *their* thing.

Fast forward to graduation. I showed up to the ceremony buzzed, and that booze fueled dozens of tears during my entry into *the real world*. Changing my major four times over three years, I studied some business, psychology, communications, and public relations, graduating as a Jen of all trades and a master of none. Still, I accomplished what I was "supposed" to do: *snag that diploma*. Teenage Jenny's purpose lied in achieving good grades and swimming fast times, but by college I strove for social appearances and male acknowledgement, all while determining my worth by how much I weighed.

By twenty-one, I established myself as a traveler, scaling success by the stamps in my passport. The more places I saw, the more like-minded people I met with an insatiable desire to wander around the world. I caught that itch, too, as flying enabled an escape which was less taboo than drug abuse. "Traveling is the healthiest addiction" was a favorite quote I saved on my Pinterest boards, justifying the urge to get up and go. Stepping off planes stimulated sensory overload. Fresh scenery secreted an amnesia sweeter than any Special K you could find at a rave, and I craved that rush at any time of the day. In my constant search for the thrill, I got high off the idea of the next flight and lost sight of the person who was enjoying the view.

...

Graduation was a blur. And so was my flight to Italy that very next day. I stepped through customs ever so cocky, thinking how cool I was for knowing what I was doing this time around. What I didn't know, however, was that everything about this time around would be much, much different.

"Ciao Jenny!" Donatella waved me down from her car with Mario and Angelica in the back seat. I did my best to reciprocate her enthusiasm, I really did. But considering I had barely slept between a week of binge drinking and this sixteen-hour travel day, I could hardly stand up straight when I stumbled off the bus from the Florence airport.

"Jenny. We are so happy you are back! I am sure you are jetlagged so feel free to sleep in tomorrow. You can start helping me with the children in the afternoon when they return from school." Donatella assured me as I sat shotgun in her silver compact car.

Ah, sleep. That sure sounded nice. I nodded in agreement, doing my best to look alert for the rest of the evening.

We stopped for ice cream before heading to Donatella's home. I tried to refuse the sweet snack as I intended to lose weight during this second stay in Italy. How could I not? It would be impossible to binge and purge while living under the surveillance of the Luis family. All I had to do was keep up with my exercise routine and mirror the meal portions of my former-model boss. I could hide my crazy for eight weeks and return home as "normal." I'd break my binging habits and slim down to my pre-Europe weight. This all made so much sense. My plan was bulletproof.

Donatella bought three scoops of chocolate gelato and I sighed in relief. She handed two cups to her children and the third to me. I waved my hand to kindly refuse.

"Jenny, eat the ice cream. You are tired and it is my treat. Please."

Well, shit.

"I am going to the market tomorrow, is there anything you need?" She asked.

"Do you have coffee at home?" Which obviously, was my only necessity.

"Of course. Anything else?" She asked.

"No thank you, Donatella."

"Any soap or shampoo?"

"I've packed all my toiletries but thank you."

"Any feminine products?" Donatella persisted.

"Oh no, I have an IUD, so I don't have a period." I said.

"You don't have a period!?" She asked.

"No, I don't have a period." I said.

"Bene. Neither do I."

When we arrived back at her house, Donatella walked me upstairs to the children's room and pointed at a twin-sized bed propped between two cribs.

"Donatella, I thought you said I would be staying next door with your mother. In my own room." I said this as softly and as passively as possible.

Donatella continued as if I never asked the question. As if we never confirmed this logistic over a Skype call when I agreed to the job at hand.

"This is your bed." Her tone shifted a couple notches stricter. "You can put your luggage underneath. Please shower and be ready for dinner in an hour." She shut the door behind her, before the room cooled down by 10 degrees.

I could not tell if I was still hungover from graduation or if my jet lag took a hold of my will to stay positive. Optimism had always been my antidote during tough times. Throughout my swimming career, I affirmed that pain is temporary, that no practice could kill me. But a somberness poured through as I stared at my new situation. Seclusion kicked in. These next few weeks would be something to "get through" as I worked to meet Donatella's expectations. I flipped through a dozen switches in my psychic circuit board, finding the positive light: I reminded myself that the opportunity would be worth it, and way more interesting than staying at home.

...

"Jenny! What do you think this is? A hotel?"

My vision focused on my Italian mother yelling from the kitchen as I wobbled down the stairs. It was 2am back home and time to get my shit together.

"I bring you into my home and you just *sleep* through everything?" Donatella shrieked.

"Sorry, Donatella... You told me to sleep off my jet lag, which I appreciate because I really needed it." I pleaded, pinning Donatella's words back onto her.

"Va bene. Be ready at 2:30 when we pick up the children at school." Still aggravated, she cooled down and left the house for groceries.

As Donatella ran errands, I ran around the cream-colored homes of Florence's suburbia. I weaved through narrow streets lined with skinny cypress trees while bumping to the same dozen songs I downloaded before my flight - an eclectic curation ranging from Shakira to Tupac. For an hour a day, I ran from my woes in a hypnotic reverie.

The shower was the only other time and place that warranted any privacy. After rinsing off from my run, I heard my name ring from downstairs.

"Jenny! Your shoes! They are terrible! Don't bring such a rancid thing into my house." Donatella yelled from the front door. Dripping, I clung onto the bath towel in silence, too embarrassed to defend myself and the stench of my sweat.

Despite all my efforts, I could do nothing right. When the children arrived back from daycare, I was never speaking enough English or saying the right thing. I couldn't even "play" to Donatella's standards, as she stepped in to criticize how I would spend too much time fixating on one game. On the fourth day of my stay, Mario had a birthday party. It was May. Mario's birthday was in January. But school was not in session during January, so Donatella made sure that Mario had a chance to celebrate his third solar return with presents and cake and ample attention just like all the other children had done so before.

After school that day, a dozen bambinos kicked and screamed through the Luis household while their mothers showed up in their finest casual wear. I wore leggings and a purple sweatshirt while arranging appetizers, under the impression I was watching the youngsters as they wrestled around. I could feel every set of the mother's eyes down my back, assuming they were commenting on my weight.

During active duty, I bussed countertops, replenished snacks, and mitigated tantrums among the toddlers, making sure the children weren't strangling each other as their moms sipped prosecco. Whenever I caught a glimpse of Mario, he was either playing alone or fighting with another kid, stripping away their toys yelling, "mio!" with roaring agitation. His lack of sociability did not surprise me in the least. But holy hell, did it stress me out.

I kept a keen eye on both the youngsters and the kitchen, surreptitiously snatching up hors d'oeuvres. The second a mom turned her padded shoulder away from the food display, I would sneak a square of pizza into my mouth, chewing slowly behind a fake smile. I was beginning to perfect my craft of stealing food and swiping chews. Despite this stealth, there was no hiding behind my ballooning cheeks.

The party hit its peak after Mario unwrapped a department store worth of toys. Once the families waved "ciao," I felt a major weight lift, despite having eaten most of the finger foods. That weight swung back when Donatella closed the door behind the last guest, firing off another round of conniving comments.

"Jenny! Look at you. Are you going to sleep? How could you wear such a thing at Mario's party? The mothers asked if you were my maid. How embarrassing." Donatella scoffed.

Defenseless, I had failed Donatella. "Nanny" was not a job title; it was an extension of her family's image.

"I'm sorry Donatella, I just wanted to be comfortable playing with the children." I sulked in my sweatshirt, wondering what was so wrong about wearing Lululemon.

Donatella sighed. "I will take the children upstairs. You can finish cleaning and get packed for tomorrow."

Friday morning, the Luis family and I huddled into their silver Mercedes Benz towards Forte dei Marmi, a chic beach town tucked between the Apuan Alps and the Tyrrhenian Sea. We drove through the brass gates of their summer home, unlocking a time capsule from the early 20th century. Soft white linens draped the golden rims of tall window frames. Classical frescos and archaic maps padded the walls of the main floor. Best of all - three flights up in a small nook, I had my own sunroom.

Every meal was al fresco on the cast iron patio set, overlooking a perfectly kept lawn enclosed by a taupe stucco fence. Donatella's pasta pomodoro slowed down time as the red wine eased the adults. This dinner was, well, *nice*. Maybe, I was getting used to nannying or maybe, the family was getting used to me.

Mr. Luis invited us into the living room, filled with cushioned wicker chairs and vintage collectables. Hanging from the wall, Mr. Luis picked up a guitar and started to strum, singing an honorable rendition of Creedence Clearwater Revival's "Have You Ever Seen The Rain?" Because he spoke little English and worked so often, I had limited interactions with Mr. Luis. But here, in his family's home, he communicated in melody imbued with meaning: *"There's a calm before the storm."*

On Saturday, the family and I rode bikes through the beach town, passing the tips of pastel pink homes, guarded by ivy-covered walls of each mansion's gate. The children's eyes got heavy, so Donatella offered to take them back to nap and suggested I continue my ride. I nearly second-guessed her offer, wondering if she would later resent giving me the break. But I took it and took off with my bike, fleeing through the manicured streets of palm trees and exotic shrubbery. Entranced by opulence, I flew high on my joy ride. My mellow return seemed to radiate throughout the Luis family that afternoon, as the rest of the day ran smoothly, without any complaints or comments from Donatella.

We spent our Sunday morning basking at a beach resort before the drive back to Florence. Striped umbrellas in white and navy lined the golden coast, where we lounged in plush beige beach chairs. While the children were in full suits and sunscreen, Donatella warned me not to let them get wet.

Mario insisted, like any toddler would, to play by the water and raced towards the waves. Donatella picked up Angelica and motioned at me to stop her son. Catching up to Mario, I took his hand and held it gently as I have an irrational fear of pulling onto a child's arm too tight and shaking a shoulder out of socket. It's called nursemaid elbow, and it's a real thing. But that was the *last* thing I needed to happen on family vacation. As we reached the shoreline, Mario slithered his hand out from mine and lunged into the water, shrieking in delight as Donatella screamed in horror. Once Mama arrived at the scene, Mario slumped into the sand, shooting out a stream of tears.

"I asked you to do one thing! *One thing!* And you can't even follow that. What good are you?" Donatella yelled.

I shook my head and looked down at Mario, who let out a giggle, gripped the sand between his fists and watched the grains dissolve back into the water. Donatella gestured towards him and again he started to cry. *Oh, I see…* This little bitch was trying to gaslight me.

"Donatella, it was an accident! He's okay. I can take him to the changing room." I said.

"Don't bother, I'll do it." Donatella handed me Angelica and scooped her other child in her arms, stomping back to our bags. As she did so, Mario's tears came to an abrupt stop as he looked up from his mother's shoulder to flash a smile that said: *"gotcha."*

At this point, there was little to say. The strain between me and Donatella was taut, and Mario sought pleasure in playing that chord. Angelica was too young to understand, and Mr. Luis was indifferent to it all. As we drove back to the suburbs in silence, I plastered a smile across my face, keen to show Donatella that she could scold me, but she would not break me.

The Luis household had no Wi-Fi. For her accounting work, Donatella operated from an internet "stick" - a device she was cautious to share and cost half of my salary for this month-long stay. Growing increasingly overwhelmed by isolation, I asked Donatella if I could bus to Florence first thing Monday morning after we took the children to daycare. She agreed as she had promised me two solo day trips in our verbal agreement.

"Thank you again Donatella!" I cheered gleefully as I exited the front door.

"Be back by 2:30" she said, emotionless.

I skipped off to the bus station, ready to revisit the first foreign city I ever fell in love with. Similarly to how I once listened to pump-up jams at a swim meet, I replayed "Hypnotize" by Biggie Smalls before my grand entrance into town. But as the doors swung open at my stop, the magic had faded. The streets, the smells and sounds were all still so lovely, still the same. I was the thing that changed, and perhaps, not in a good way. I expected the sense of wonder to ignite in me like it did in August 2013. Instead, I showed up at my old apartment like an ex-girlfriend creeping on her long-lost lover's address.

Hmm… What was off? What needed to be fixed for me to be happy in Florence once again? Obviously, the answer was ice cream. Knowing just the place, I popped inside Gelateria de Neri and snapped selfies with my sweet treat. Lingering in a Wi-Fi zone outside a cafe, I uploaded the pics to social media and waited for the likes to pour in. Refresh. Refresh. Refresh. *Notification!* Someone commented: "I'm so jealous."

Jealous? Of what? Of Donatella's verbal abuse and my mental obsessions around food?

Reading with dejection, I felt fraudulent, framing au pair life as a glamorous destination. This employment was draining the life out of me. There was certainly *nothing* to be jealous about.

While my deceiving post evoked a shallow sense of connection, I needed to procure internet access at the Luis home. Using my first week's stipend, I bought a cheap, low-speed internet chip before returning to the burbs. That evening, I uploaded photos on Facebook, which reaped a response shortly after I hit publish.

@Audra Allen: "Hey, I just walked by there!"

The Facebook notification caught me off guard but was well received. Audra Allen was a soft-spoken acquaintance of whom I had known since middle school. Without hesitation, I messaged Audra about grabbing a drink over the upcoming weekend, figuring I'd coordinate with my live-in mother the next morning. I shut my laptop in relief. I was five thousand miles from home, yet a piece - or a person - of familiarity was now within reach.

The Tuscan sunshine woke me up before my alarm the next morning, promising a bright day ahead. After dropping the children off at daycare, I galloped to gangster rap while Donatella picked up groceries. We arrived back to the house simultaneously, so I lent a hand to keep my Italian mother's mood at bay and my runner's high intact. As I walked towards her silver Opel to help with the groceries, she held up her hand to protest:

"Jenny no! You're dirty! Go inside and clean off." She shooed me away and I headed inside to shower.

I decided to fill the bathtub, however, compelled to completely submerge my body. Silence awaited me beneath the water, only as long as I could hold my breath.

Watching the maelstrom spiral down the drain, the gurgling sound of water became drowned by a scream.

"JENNY!"

'How could I have already messed up?' I thought as I scurried out of the tub and threw on clothes. She waited for me in the kitchen, waiving my used coffee mug in the air.

"I let you into my home, you trash it with your awful shoes... Now *this*! Che schifo, you are worthless!" As my bare feet crossed into kitchen territory, she claimed her space, stepping in front of my face, shaking her bony fists while piercing her eyes through my skull.

"Why do you run? You think it will make you thin? You will never be thin. You are a fat, ugly American. You have gotten fatter since the day I met you and your birth control has messed with your hormones." Her voice wavered as her cheeks blushed with blood. She took a breath for the next blow and persisted.

"You are not the same person I hired last fall. I hired a beautiful, American girl and I have brought back a monster." Her heels hovered off the tiled floor, her body now towering over mine.

Frozen in fear, my eyes welled, jaw shut tight. But I would not allow her to scrutinize me like this, my pride had to prevail. A single tear of remorse streamed down my face before I wiped it away and steeled my nerves.

"Donatella..." I cleared my throat and matched her daunting stare.

"I apologize about the mug. But I won't apologize for running or my weight. It is a shame for you to say this. It is a shame you must condemn my body to beat me down. But the biggest shame is hearing you call me a monster and still allowing me to watch your children. You're right, though. I have changed, and I will no longer stand for this mistreatment. I'm sorry but I don't trust you, and I'm afraid I'll have to leave."

My voice shook, but I stuck up for myself. Donatella could call me fat, ugly, and stupid. She could accuse my birth control for my behavior - despite having inserted the IUD *before* I even met her. But to call me a monster, to depict my nature as deplorable and still want me to work as her nanny was ludicrous. It was abuse.

111

"You won't get away with this!" She trembled with anger.

"You can't leave me. You can't leave our family like this." Donatella was now in full panic mode, wailing around, trying to seize back her power.

"I'm sorry, Donatella. I don't feel safe." I said, holding my guard as I returned to my room, where I shut the door behind me to break down and cry.

Never had I felt so humiliated. I had been called a slut, a quitter, and an addict in the past, accepting these insults as reverberations of my actions. But the words "worthless" and "monster" shot through my core. I might have slept with my ex's friend and gone to great lengths to buy a half ounce of weed. I might have been selfish, even a fiend. But I never meant any harm, and I wasn't about to let some stranger I met off the internet treat me like this. Though to her, I was a stranger from the internet, too, in Italy on her dime, under her roof. I was stranger, welcomed into a strange home, now desperate to get the fuck out.

With my newly purchased Wi-Fi chip, I messaged my mom and Audra in distress, pleading for a plane ticket home and a place to crash for the time being. Audra offered up her couch without question. However, my mom wasn't too happy to bail me out of this purgatory I had put myself in, but she wasn't going to let her only daughter suffer under the scrutiny of another mother.

I typed silently in my room and considered sneaking out of the house when Donatella picked up the children from daycare, but when my own mother tried altering my return flight from her end, Donatella received an email from the airlines and burst into the bedroom.

"You are trying to *leave me?!* After all I have done for you? I paid for your flights. I have paid for your food. I have given you a place to stay. For you to desert our family after you made a commitment is to steal from me. Mario and Angelica have drawn attached to you. For you to run away like this will cause *moral damage* to my children."

I stared up at Donatella, contemplating the "moral damage" I would cast upon the toddlers. Luckily for Mario and Angelica, they were only getting a week of Jenny Martin. Imagine how damaged those kids would end up if they were raised by a monster like me...

Donatella saw my opened suitcase and demanded I join her to pick up the kids from daycare. "How dare you betray my family like this. We have had many nannies in the past, but no one has been as lazy as you." Her knuckles paled as she clawed onto the wheel.

There was no use in defending myself. No use in pointing out her weak retention rate or inquiring about the litany of anonymous nannies. Meditating in the passenger seat, I let her words pass over me like a strong wind. She could ruffle me up, but she would not push me down. What felt like an hour later, we pulled up to daycare.

"Mario! Angelica!" Donatella swept her children into the car just like any other afternoon.

"Ciao bambini... Jenny has decided to leave us today. Aren't you sad?"

Mario shot us a delightfully confused stare. For three years old, he was quite the actor.

"Mama?" Mario looked at his mother for validation.

"Si, Mario, Jenny is leaving. She does not want to be with us any longer." Donatella stared into her son's eyes, who noticed her hint and started to cry.

I sat speechless, shocked, and impotent. It was only a matter of time before Donatella would source another pitiful thing to hire as her sitter. However, I was checked out and could cross "au pair" off my bucket list. I pursued this position because of my adoration for children, for cultural immersion, and for sheer experience. What I received was more than what I had asked for, more than I could manage.

In summary, I agreed to stay eight weeks with the Luis family and resigned after nine days. Any time longer would have sacrificed my sanity and so I jumped ship. I felt like a failure, but at least I was free.

Donatella barked at me as my suitcase flopped down her stairs. "You have caused my children moral damage." She repeated from the living room, maintaining a cheerful tone in her voice to keep her children from startling.

"This will all come back to you. The pain you are causing my family will all come back to you. What comes around, goes around Jenny."

Before I closed the front door behind me, I turned towards the stranger I had met on the internet one final time. "Certainly Donatella, something we can finally agree on."

After this Italian job fiasco, I contemplated the law of karma. While I'll never know the fate of Donatella Luis following my leave, I found myself in a string of fortunate events soon after.

Back in middle school, Audra Allen and I had a few classes together. We were never close friends, but we had a kind correspondence. This courtesy built an unspoken trust between us two, which granted me a couch to sleep on when I found myself stranded in Italy. What I'm trying to say is, be nice to people. Especially in middle school. Because you never know when you'll need a couch to sleep on when you find yourself stranded in Italy.

Audra and I caught up effortlessly, with much to share about the past four years (let alone the past four hours) of our lives. Audra was finishing an apprenticeship with a local artist, extending her stay in Florence from the typical semester cycle. By the time I arrived, a new wave of students had settled into Audra's apartment. When I asked her what she thought of her new tenants, the light in her eyes started to dim.

"Let's just say they're not the brightest bunch." She said, exhausted.

"The other week, and let me be clear, these girls have been here for a month now – my roommate was complaining about her cell phone service, so I told her to go to the Vodafone by the Duomo... She asked, 'the *what*?' and I said, 'the Duomo...'"

"THE DUOMO?" I reiterated.

"Yes, Jenny! My roommates still don't know what the Duomo is, nor do they care. I'm over it." Audra's shoulders slumped as she shook her head.

The Basilica de Santa Maria del Fiore, or the Duomo, is so grandeur and central to Florence, that ignoring its presence is comparable to asking about the pretty pyramid structure glistening over the Seine River in Paris. Audra was clearly in distress over her new roommates, counting down the days until she reunited with her family back in Kansas City.

I asked to crash for five nights until my budget flight to Amsterdam, a trip I booked before the nanny fall-out, to meet up with backpacking buddies and then make my way home. My short stay in Audra's apartment didn't seem to bother her roommates when they checked out the 'new girl,' seeing I had already created a corner of my things beside the couch. Though I couldn't help but hear a murmur between the thin Florentine walls. Luckily, this posse packed up for a weekend trip to Venice the first morning of my stay, leaving space for me and Audra to breathe... and booze for the night.

I, Jennifer Martin, am fully aware that I am an enabler, enticing indulgence from any surrounding associates. Audra, however, is a modest drinker and yet our "casual night out" quickly turned into a full-fledged affair. The two of us wide-eyed girlies managed to track in a couple American soldiers back to the apartment, letting them crash before they caught the train to their military base in Pisa the next morning. When I awoke, the guys were gone, but they left the roommate's beds discombobulated. I too, woke up looking like a mess, though on the couch, brain dead, nursing my headache by scrolling through my phone. As I opened Snapchats, I wondered why my friends back home were online at such strange hours. I tiptoed into Audra's room with sleepy eyes, telling her how

115

odd it was that people were snapping me at work when it was midnight back home.

"Uh… Jenny. It's 6pm. Not 6am. You slept through the entire day." She giggled.

Ah. That explains everything.

"Oh… Well then. It's time for dinner!"

Audra and I bought a spread of cheese and cured meats and returned to her living room to eat. As we chewed on ciabatta, her roommates walked in. They arrived a day earlier than expected, before we had a chance to change the sheets and erase any evidence of our male guests' impromptu visit.

"Yea hi, Audra? Can we have a roommate meeting? Like, right now?" The alpha female of the wolf pack stood center of the four women, lined up with crossed arms and lifted noses sniffing for drama.

"We've decided as roommates that she can't stay. She can sleep here tonight but needs to leave in the morning." Barked the alpha dog, avoiding eye contact with me.

I laughed in disbelief. This whole scene was so stagy and savage. I mean… plenty of strangers had slept in those beds before them and like, come on, bitch, I have a name.

"There are hotels in Florence. She can go somewhere else." The alpha summoned the rest of the litter back to her room to do what I can only imagine was gossip about this conundrum. Audra and I ran back to her room to do the same.

"I hate this!" Audra cried. "A roommate decision? How could they say such a thing without including me…? I lived here before them and now they are going to decide on who gets to come through the doors? I'm asking my parents if they can get me a hotel for my last week. I can't take this anymore." She pushed back her silky black hair and buried her face in her hands. Audra was not one for drama. And while we were both at fault for letting some dudes crash in her roommate's beds, the soldiers simply *slept*. We had every intention of washing their sheets... we just lost track of time.

We sat in Audra's bed, comforting one another. I tried not to panic as booking a hotel was not an option. Neither was asking my parents to wire me money, considering how pissed they were when they paid for my flight home.

Just as I was losing hope, Audra received a Facebook message from one of her sorority sisters. Audra's friend Lexi had just landed in Florence for her summer semester and found out that her roommate had dropped out of the program at the last minute. Meaning, Lexi had an extra bed, and offered it to me.

Altruism saved me from the streets that week, showing me that sometimes generosity does not demand immediate reciprocity. Good fortune returns in divine timing. My angels, Audra and Lexi, brought me in for reasons I'll never know, but they trusted me and wanted to keep a fellow Midwestern gal safe overseas. And though I was dumb broke that week, I tried to pay things forward with positivity and – *cheesy spoiler alert* - the gift of presence.

Karma is less about "good vs. bad," but more so an input and output of action kinda thing. Thus, with every stride, karma kept showing up. With two nights to spare in Florence, my study abroad babe, Brooklyn, just happened to be in town with her family, who happily adopted me as one of their own. Brooklyn's warm, generous parents took care of me and the bill for every meal we spent together. During the last dinner, we passed vino rosso across our table at Osteria Santo Spirito, dining on the cobblestone patio beneath twinkling string lights.

"Jenny, what has Italy taught you this time around?" asked Brooklyn's dad. I looked up from my pillows of potato gnocchi, still bubbling in its skillet, releasing an aroma of gorgonzola and truffle oil.

"Hmm..." I swirled the red wine in my glass, watching the legs drip down as I contemplated my answer.

"I learned that I'm guilty of following my desires… rather my gut. Like, I had a feeling Donatella was a little crazy, but I wanted a ticket back to Italy. Though I don't regret anything. Because no matter where I go, I always find someone who is willing to help when things - and people - get a little crazy." I took a sip of my wine and leaned over to Brooklyn, sitting next to me.

Brooklyn swung her arm around my shoulder.

"You're always taken care of Jenny." She said as she squeezed me.

For those 48 hours, my belly stayed full, my heart light and my wallet completely untouched. I was extremely grateful for Brooklyn and her parents; and for the first time on that trip, I felt safe.

...

Last stop: Holland. Where I'd meet up with college friends backpacking for the summer. However, those homies would arrive a day after me, so I reached out to a Dutch girl I met from my Italian semester to see if she could hang. Although she was out of the country, she connected me with her friend Anna who was studying in Amsterdam. Anna - with zero obligation - spent the afternoon with me, taking me to popular *pleins*, indulged in a "coffee shop" toke, and even bought my dinner to disprove the stereotype that the Dutch are cheap. We ate fries smothered in mayonnaise alongside the Amstel River, where a string of colonial Dutch buildings lined up in brick, brown, and red, with white window frames and pointed gambrels. While picking through my *patat* snack from a paper cone, I realized it had been days since I bought my own meal. When sweet, sweet Anna said goodbye at the bus stop, she gave me a hug and wished me luck. I held my tears until I hopped into my seat and let out a blissful sigh. After everything that had happened in the past week, I felt like the luckiest girl in the world.

What I experienced in Holland only further reinforced my karmic observances: when you are kind, kindness reciprocates. But kindness and karma won't cover your broke, dumb ass when your connecting flight into America has been delayed due to a storm. I had $35 in my account and a few singles in my wallet when I touched down in Miami after a hectic layover in Madrid. At this point, I was so emotionally dilapidated that sleeping in the airport might have sent me into cardiac arrest, an anxiety attack, or worse, a raging bitch. With my final five dollars, I bought a Snickers bar at an airport kiosk and summoned the strength to call my mother for a money wire.

"Mom, my flight is delayed until tomorrow. Can you *please* send me some money for a hotel? My body is in so much pain, the jet lag is making me nauseous. I just need a bed for tonight." I cried.

"I'm about to order dinner, I'll have to call you back." *Click*

Ouch.

But alas, Mrs. Martin wired $100 into my account, which was enough for a sleazy airport motel. I prayed to stay clear of traffickers and bed bugs. I prayed for my headache to go away. But mostly, I prayed to give thanks to my parents, Brooklyn's parents, Audra, Anna, and their parents, who raised such wonderful daughters. I prayed that the next few weeks would go much smoother than the previous two, and that my new life on cruise ships would open an adventurous, *affluent* chapter of my life.

Gallery Girl

I woke up in my musty motel room under a stiff, quilted comforter. A hazy glow came from the windows which were dripping in condensation; yesterday's storm made for a humid morning in Miami. Skies were clear for take-off, and I was cleared of all the trouble I started in Europe... or so I thought.

Two flights later, my brother Matt picked me up from the Kansas City Airport with a weed pen in hand, offering me a rip. As I inhaled, he chuckled:

"Dude. Not gonna lie, Mom and Dad are pissed at you."

I started coughing as he turned on the highway.

"What? Why?" I looked at my brother, who was simply a blonder version of my dad. Blue eyes and strong jawlines, with strong bodies they have never had a problem maintaining despite their diet rich in red meat and ample sweets.

"I mean, you just flew to Europe without having enough money to make it back." Matt sighed with a slight smile; he knew I'd absorb all ridicule during dinner. He turned towards a divey barbeque joint, one with a cartoon pig on the restaurant's sign. Matt was right, I didn't have a backup plan with the nanny gig, and I didn't have enough saved in case shit hit the fan...which it totally did.

As Matt and I entered the restaurant, I spotted my parents in a burgundy booth. They lifted their noses from the menus the second they heard the bell chime from the front door. "Alright, Red." My dad motioned at my mom to shuffle out of their seats to give me an obligatory embrace.

The four of us sat in silence. Our eyes played tennis from the menu to me, to my parents back to me, then out of bounds to Matt, who was texting his girlfriend. No one spoke until the waitress dropped off our baskets.

"Mmm... barbeque. How I missed it!" I decided to break the ice.

The past fortnight, I had been maxing out my dollar with street foods or eating out on another's dime. Communal meals and a lack of funds prevented binges - which prevented purges - and so, I considered myself cured.

"Jenny..." My dad was here for burnt ends, not my bologna.

"After prancing off to Italy like that, I'm not so sure ships are in your best interest." he said sternly.

I swallowed a bite of an onion ring, collecting my response.

"But dad, Galleries at Sea is a global company. The average entry rate is $700 a week, without *any* expenses! I'm not watching some Italian woman's toddlers. I'm selling art. It's a sales job. That's what you wanted for me, wasn't it?" While trying to sell him on this idea, all I wanted was to buy his approval.

"I suppose it is sales. Let's just hope they send you somewhere nice and warm." He sighed. My mind was made. No use lecturing now. I'm a Martin, and we Martins do what we want to do. *This Martin* goes wherever she wants to go. Though in this case, I would go wherever the contract would take me.

"Yea." My mom added, "Let's hope you don't go to *Alaska.*"

...

A month and some change later, I'm dressed in a red power dress and white kitten heels, with straightened hair and a fresh face of makeup, primed for my final day of training in Miami. After a week of written tests, artist presentations, role plays and Q&A panels, it was time to graduate and receive our placements. Fifty associates from South Africa, Romania, The UK, Canada, and a handful of other nations gathered in a vast event space to find out where we would be stationed for the next six months. Our silver-haired sales trainer stood in a black suit on center stage, announcing everyone's assignments, one-by-one.

"Jennifer Martin... signing on as art associate on the Queen Pearl. Point of call: Vancouver, British Columbia."

Hearing my name through the speakers, I shot up from my row of chairs and headed towards the stage to shake the trainer's hand and grab my welcome packet.

I'd fly to Vancouver that night and board The Queen Pearl first thing in the morning. From there, the ship would sail north for its itinerary around... *Alaska.* High off the promise of adventure, I sauntered through Canadian customs that evening, thrilled to add a new stamp in my passport. Besides the flight, Galleries at Sea had not fronted any other expense, but booked me a room for a hefty $250 dollars in downtown Vancouver. With double digits in my bank account, I lugged my two suitcases up and down the rolling hills of the port city, knocking on hotel doors to check for subsidized rates.

"Hi, hello I'm looking for a room tonight. I start my first job tomorrow, and I'm afraid my company didn't set me up in a room I could afford. I don't have much, so I was hoping to fill any vacancies." I stared straight into the soul of the middle-aged clerk, sighing to signal exhaustion and showing him that my American phone didn't have a signal. This man looked as tired as I did, considering it was midnight.

"Sure, dear. I can't have you looking for a bed this late at night in the city. I can put you up in a single for fifty." said the clerk.

"Thank you!" I sighed in relief. I could have hugged him - kissed him! But I refrained.

"You don't know how much this means to me." I affirmed as he led me up a clamorous elevator and to my door.

"Here's your key. You must have an angel watching you, girl. You caught me just as I was heading out for the night. Good luck with your new job." He dropped the key in my hand and headed down the hallway.

"Thank you." I said as he left.

I looked at the key and whispered, *"thank you."* I had an angel watching over me indeed.

At 6am the next day, I suited up in a royal, floral pencil skirt and a cream-colored blouse, complete with those white kitten heels and fine-tipped eye liner. Striding a good kilometer in my pointed shoes, I rolled my belongings across Vancouver's West End to Coal Harbour, where hordes of red, white, and blue tugboats lined the port, and half a dozen cruise liners scattered across broad cement docks. I followed signs for the Queen Pearl and headed towards her thousand-foot-long majesty.

The salty air from the Pacific Coast brushed my skin for the first time as I entered a week of firsts. My first day of work for my first job out of college. (Discounting my stint with Donatella.) The Queen Pearl would be my first steps on a cruise ship, getting my first taste of what it meant to travel for work. Not only would I churn a steady paycheck, I lived rent free. I gained full access to buffets and gyms. I had no water or energy bill. Beer at the crew bar started at $1, and there was no need to shop for clothes as the sliver of a closet I had in my cabin could not possibly squeeze in another pencil skirt. My parents thought I was foolish for taking a job on cruise ships, but I thought of myself as clever. However clever, I would still need to prove myself to my first ever full-time boss.

Dante Coetzee was a formidable, burly man with porcelain skin and sleepy blue eyes. His dark, gelled hair and wide smile fit him like a prom king that never let go of his glory days. I could not pin down how old he was, maybe thirty-five or so, but I could tell that this job had aged him.

Dante greeted me in the ship's health clinic once the nurses cleared me from my screening. Immediately, he scanned my professional attire with great discernment.

Is my skirt too short? It hits at my knees! I thought nervously. Dante sized me up, checking for signs of incompetency, idiocy, and the ill intent of wanting this job for anything other than money.

"Hello, Jennifer. Welcome to the Queen Pearl. I don't expect you to know much or sell much but I do expect you to work hard and listen to what I tell you to do. We'll have a team meeting in the gallery at 6pm tonight. That should give you some time to finish orientation and settle into your cabin. Charlotte is your cabin mate. She will meet you here and show you to your quarters before muster at 4pm."

"What's a mu-" I cocked my head as I spoke in a high pitch.

"I must be going. See you at four." Dante looked annoyed, like he had important matters to tend to, adjusted his stance to puff his chest and left.

Over stimulated on this day of "firsts," I was too aroused for Dante to intimidate me. I too had important matters to tend too, like how find my cabin... or get anywhere for that matter.

A short, curly haired blonde in her late twenties from Virginia begrudgingly introduced herself. "I'm Charlotte."

Charlotte had been working under Dante for five months after two years in the company. Her metal frames hunched over her curvy nose, with her squinty eyes observing me through thick glass.

"So... this is your first contract? Good luck. Dante is good... really good at his job. Do what he says, and you should be ok." She sighed.

I should be ok? I'm a god-damn millennial. I better be thriving. I thought.

Charlotte led us to deck six, where we stopped at a bar lounge rimmed in chestnut oak, coated in gold and royal rugs, and filled with evergreen furniture.

"This is the Executive Lounge. Get familiar - you'll be spending the next six months in this place." Charlotte and I scanned the ornate room decorated with plush club chairs and wooden cocktail tables glowing with bronze sconces. Theater seating and spotlights drew our eyes towards center stage, where I envisioned myself holding the mic:

"Ladies and Gentlemen!"

Charlotte snapped me back: "Let's keep moving."

Past the Executive Lounge, I followed Charlotte up to the Promenade deck and into the gallery before I stopped dead in sheer excitement.

Peter Max! Romero Britto! Is that... a limited edition of... no... it can't be... Joan Miro!

The studio lights highlighted dozens of artists I had meticulously studied over the past month, inventing parasocial relationships with each one to develop my understanding of their work. And here we were, all hanging out as they hung in front of me. It was like meeting your favorite celebrities for the first time… at a wax museum.

The most popular and profitable artist the Queen Pearl kept in her collection was Peter Max, a pop-art expressionist recognized for his psychedelic styles from the 1960's and 1970's. As an art associate, I became very familiar with Mr. Max. My main objective was marketing in the middle of the bustling Promenade deck, asking guests to 'Pick the Price of the Peter Max, whilst registering them for our free auctions. An alluring painting would catch a passenger's eye, and I would work to transfer that attention into a potential sale, up to six hours a day.

In the gallery, another art associate sat erect behind a desk, cutting raffle tickets for 'Pick the Price' by hand. Alice from South Africa lifted her head to greet me with a warm smile. Her tight blonde ringlets bounced against her ivory skin. The way Alice said, "hello, Jennifer," was ever so soothing. "Welcome to ship life."

"Please, call me Jenny" I smiled back.

"Ah! Jenny!" An unfamiliar voice rushed past behind me. I turned around a little too fast, nearly smacking my gallery director, Maria Popa, in the face as she reached for my hand. I held my breath, startled by Maria's curt grip.

"Ciao, Jenny. We are so happy to have another associate on the team!" Maria's tone was sincere yet snappy. Her raw energy left me speechless as my eyes dilated to soak her in, unsure of what to say and do next.

"Look at those big eyes, Jenny! Be careful with those babe," said Maria.

Maria Popa had a stern confidence about her. She was a Romanian woman in her late twenties, maybe early thirties. It was hard to tell given her dyed black hair, layers of makeup and affinity for cigarettes. A diligent businesswoman, Maria's extensive stiletto collection added inches to her petite frame. Gregarious, Maria could talk to anyone. She took pleasure in weaving various European expressions amidst the four languages she fluently spoke.

"Andiamo, bambini!" Maria summoned the three blonde associates through the flood doors connecting the gallery to the ship's chapel. Maria pulled up a beige chair from a stack against a beige wall and directed us to follow suit along the beige and brown carpet. Just as I reached for a seat, Dante peered through the double-winged doors, suited up and freshly groomed.

"Afternoon, ladies."

The room shrank as I took my seat, and a blur of beige started to swallow me whole.

Now, I am a pretty smart person. But at the beginning of any new job, I'm regretfully reticent, learning the hard way that there *is* such a thing as asking a dumb question. In this meeting, I sat looking more pretty than I did smart.

"Let's make this a good cruise, ladies." Dante began lecturing. "We are close to leading the fleet, but we are still two thousand behind the Coral Captiva. We may have hit our sales target the past three cruises, but I will not settle for anything less than $100,000 this week. We need to push the premium bids and hand out at least five hundred more raffle tickets for "Pick The Pri…""

Blah, blah, blah… When will we be in Alaska? I was hoping he would go over the itinerary, not just numbers. Dante continued reviewing sales from the previous cruise, though my lack of reference made it difficult to follow.

"Popa!" Dante yelled, with Maria sitting inches away from his feet.

"How many mixed medias did you sell last week?" Dante asked.

"Four. Two of the Rafael Angels, one Castillo and one Antoni Meade." Maria said without hesitation.

The Angels? Castillo? Antoni Meade? These artists weren't mentioned in my training! I quickly snapped out of my daydream of dog sledding with Siberian huskies down a glacier in Juneau.

"What are the Angels?" I asked sheepishly.

The room died down, and four startled faces looked my way.

"Asseblief!" Dante roared, throwing one hand in the air.

"I told them not to send me another American." He mumbled, loud enough for us all to hear.

I turned to Charlotte, not sure what to do.

"Those artists weren't on our study guide." I pointed out.

"Ha!" Dante patted his stomach.

"A study guide won't prepare you for much in life, let alone this job." He chuckled and grabbed hold of the brass doorknob of the chapel.

"That's enough for now. Get some rest before Pick the Price. You all look tired." He swung open the door towards the gallery and stepped out.

My coworkers dispersed like all the confidence I had conjured up from training. It was day one of a six-month contract. The Queen Pearl began closing its gates to head north towards Ketchikan, and I sure as hell wasn't going anywhere soon.

Charlotte showed me to our cabin, a hiccup of space located three decks below sea level. "This is technically not our assigned cabin. We are supposed to be one level up with gift shop and photog, in rooms with carpet and a desk. The rooms are small either way."

Charlotte inserted her key card and pressed down on the steel handle. I entered and put my two suitcases against the bunk bed, filling up half the room.

"Once you empty your luggage, you can fit them under my bed. But that can wait. It's time for muster drill."

Charlotte and I grabbed our orange life vests hanging on the door and left our crammed little quarters. Going into this contract, I knew crew life would have its quirks devoid of glamour. Still, through my forced smile, I cringed. I recalibrated. This is what I signed up for and this is what I wanted...*wasn't it?*

The doors to the sixth deck led us through a portal between working crew members and paying guests. Dozens of northern North Americans wobbled through the gates, catching their "sea legs" towards the gallery and into the chapel for the mandatory safety drill. Maria handed me a gadget to scan key cards of the Canadian and American adults huddled around me like yellow minions speaking gibberish.

"Oo ho lo ho…. We are Platinum Members… ha ho" I scanned the chrome card of a silver-haired man in a large tee-shirt that said: "CANCUN."

Hordes of humans shuffled into their seats while a remaining few filed along the walls, disappointed to have to wait another half hour before the bar opened. I surveyed their faces. Some looked hungry, some looked drunk. Most looked like they were waiting for a rollercoaster to drop, while one couple looked like they would kick it any minute. After all, the majority of the Queen Pearl demographic was Caucasian, affluent and old. *

My editor advised I use the word "senior" for inclusivity and well, not sound so ignorant and immature. But as a twenty-something telling this story, that's exactly what I was. Funny, how at my age everyone seems to be either young or old. And that the youth wastes so much money and energy preventing the inevitable, human process of aging.

"Ladies and Gentlemen, may I have your attention please..." The muster drill commenced.

Fifty faces glazed over as Maria and I demonstrated how to fasten a life jacket. Minutes later, the room fizzled out and I headed to my first shift for 'Pick the Price' one deck down at the Promenade.

I shadowed Charlotte for the first few days as Dante didn't want me screwing up or missing any opportunities of catching the *whales*. That is, a prospect worth ten-fold of the average lead. I had a great deal of sales terminology to learn in a short amount of time, from whales and washes, leads and low-hanging fruit, to identifying the gatekeeper in a relationship, and the art of mirroring. Luckily, mirroring came second nature to me. Mirroring example:

A couple walks up to the Statue of Liberty painting.

Guest: "Oh! Honey! Isn't that pretty?"

Me: "Ah, yes, quite pretty, isn't it?"

Guest: Asks questions with a slight head tilt

Me: Answers questions with a slight head tilt

Guest: (Points at my tag: JENNIFER, USA, ART GALLERY)

"What are you doing working on ships as an American?"

Me: "What are *you* doing cruising for vacation as an American?"

I bit my tongue every time a guest investigated my motives for becoming a crew member, as if such a title was designated for the nationalities they deemed of as 'lesser.' Too often, guests asked about my plans for the future or if I went to college, invalidating my intelligence and integrity because I worked on ships. They wondered why a pretty, white girl like me would waste my youth and live below deck to serve the Jones's from the dry land.

My undercurrent of resentment was unfair to these innocuous inquiries as these folks were on island time with little on the mind. Though I did find it funny how often people asked which way the front of the ship was when I stood next to a large window facing the waves.

"Ah, the front of the ship, sir?" I'd reiterate as I looked out the window, watching the current pass us.

"Yea, that's what I said." The guest would grumble, as if in some kind of hurry.

I'd lift a hand towards the window to hint at the waves, then guided it up the hallway.

"You're headed in the right direction, welcome aboard." I'd reply.

I swear, you could be a surgeon with 20 years of practice under your belt, but once the Tommy Bahamas pop on, all commonsense washes away with one Mai Tai. I understand that people don't go on vacation to *think* and that I worked in hospitality to *serve*. But when I was asked if the crew members slept on board, I couldn't help but respond, "No, we take a helicopter to a hotel in Canada and fly back every morning to the next port."

My sarcasm might make me chuckle, but it usually came back to bite me. Between my 'Pick the Price' shifts, I stood nervously in the gallery as Dante audited every interaction I had with potential buyers. Quite soon, he advised me to charm the guests and hand them off to him because clearly, I didn't know what I was doing. He was the toxic dance mom peering through the crowd of my recital, ready to watch me fall. Under his pressure, I tripped over my own feet. When that dance was over, the entire team felt the burden of my mistakes.

"Popa!" Dante yelled for Maria, implying that the rest of the art team line up for a lecture.

The four females took a seat around Dante in the chapel once more, whipping out notepads in the sea of beige.

"We haven't made any sales tonight, so someone *please* give me some good news. Alice, what did you come up with?" Dante took a caramel cushioned chair and collapsed in his seat. My head perked up. *Leads? Crap!* I had been busy deflecting the guest's questions about my personal life and failed to gather intel from Pick the Price.

"I have Mr. and Mrs. Robins in cabin 4021. They bought two mixed medias last year on a different fleet," said sweet Alice with slight hesitation.

"Is that all? The Robins with two mixed medias?" asked Dante.

"Yes," whispered Alice.

"Marvelous," sighed Dante.

He shot a look at Charlotte.

"I have the Millers of cabin 2340 and the Kleins of cabin 1230 and…."

Charlotte was clearly the kid in school who raised their hand at every question, even after the teacher suggested: *"does anyone else want to answer who hasn't yet?"*

Then it was my turn.

"Ha, well… totally forgot about taking notes as I'm still, you know, soaking it all in. *But* I did build rapport with a couple who went to my alma mater!"

I laughed at myself since no one else seemed to find my lack of preparation as cute as I did.

"Jenny! What did they bring you on for? I specifically asked the gallery to stop bringing me girls and they brought me another *American* girl.

The trainers assured me you were top of your class, and I expect to see results." Dante's voice reverberated through my bones.

I almost said it, but I refrained. The two words people, mostly women, misuse and excuse themselves with all too often. A phrase you might hear when you bump into someone when it was entirely your fault. But unless you are at fault for something and you mean it, there is no reason to ever say: "I'm sorry."

Instead of apologizing for not meeting expectations, I looked Dante in the eyes and said: "Understood."

Once Dante released us at 10pm that night, I rushed to my cabin, closed the curtains on my top half of the bunk and wept into my pillow. How could someone be so crass to someone they just met? Yesterday, I graduated top of my training class, feeling on top of the world. Now I was drowning, about to take the ship down with me.

My phone's alarm blared under my pillow. Disoriented, I reminded myself that I was on the top bunk of a cabin in a boat. That I chose this life and that meant sacrificing a nightstand. I did my darn best not to startle Charlotte as I changed into the sports bra and running shorts I had tucked in the corner of my bed the night before, slid down the aluminum ladder and headed to the gym.

Fresh on the boat, I assured myself I would maintain healthy routines during ship life. And what a life it was with access to the guest gym, a privilege granted to a fraction of crew members of a certain rank, so long as we remained identifiable as crew members by always wearing name tags. Overlooking the waves from the front of the ship, I ran five files before 7am, a modest distance considering I ran in the Miami heat every afternoon of training, while eating little from the stress of studying. This slimmed me down a couple pounds from my most recent Euro trip, and I was determined to keep on shrinking.

At 7:30am I met Maria, Charlotte, and Alice in the Executive Lounge to set up the auction. Charlotte directed an additional staff of porters to assemble carpeted trollies as Maria filled them with artwork. Alice went for the easels, and I tried to not look like a total dipshit.

"Bumblebee!" Maria yelled across the lounge.

Who, me?

"You! Bumblebee! With the big eyes! Take the trollies near the stage, empty the art, and come back for more. Okie dokie?"

Okie dokie.

I had already built up a sweat from my morning run, ignorant of the exertion I would endure on this first full day at sea. We set up over one hundred art works in an hour, weaving easels in meticulous angles to showcase as much merchandise as possible. The room glistened. I too, was ready to shine.

Three hours later, after another "Pick the Price" shift, Dante sat the team down in the Executive Lounge for a pep-talk before the auction. Except it was less pep and more threat. A threat-talk, I should say.

"How are we feeling today, ladies?" Dante directed the question my way. I perked up and adjusted my blouse printed with blue anchors, totally on brand.

"Great! I went on a run, reviewed my study guide, and had a productive Pick the Price. I'm ready to go!" I announced.

Maria, Charlotte, and Alice looked at me like I had just admitted I was wildly hungover. I winced, starkly sober.

"We cannot waste our energy at the gym! Conserve it to sell. Trust me, you'll get your exercise on the floor." Dante roared.

O, crap. Did I do something wrong? Since when is exercise reprimanded? Didn't Dante understand that exercising generates energy? I suppressed a surge of tears that welled behind my eyes. Why scrutinize me *now* when I was in high spirits? If this was a pep-talk, what would a *"you gon' fucked up"* talk look like?

Dismissed, the team took their positions for the auction, and I stayed sulking in my seat. Maria turned to me with a strict voice and motherly concern.

"Jenny, I don't want to hear it. If you need to run, run. But don't let anyone hear it. Don't let Dante know about what you do outside of work, ok?"

"Ok." I said, wiping a tear from my cheek.

"Good. Now focus on talking to as many people as possible today. Ask questions and find leads. Don't worry about the sale, just keep people interested in the art. No go on, Bumblebee. *Buzz!*"

She wouldn't say so for another few weeks, but Maria believed in me. And while she spoke many languages, this nickname said it all: *I was going to be ok.*

"Ladies and Gentlemen!" Dante grabbed the gavel in one hand, the mic in the other. Between Dante and our team, he could cut through flesh with one pensive stare. Between Dante and the audience, he could sell art to the blind. His playful banter on stage and South African accent allured any guest on the sixth deck into the Executive Lounge. Once Dante started the bid, he blew everyone away.

Like the captive audience, my attention drew towards the stage. That was until I felt Charlotte's eyes peer at me through her glasses.

"Don't just stand there!" She mouthed as her palms spread with an annoyed jerk. Nervously, I leaned over a couple sipping their complimentary champagne, awkwardly kneeling beside the wife as she lifted her flute.

"What do we think? I asked, gesturing at the stage.

The wife nearly choked on her bottom-shelf bubbly.

"Fine, thank you." She coughed.

I had worked at Ann Taylor long enough to pick up what they were putting down: *We're just looking, thanks. No intention to buy. Only here to pass the time until Bingo starts at 2pm.*

I avoided another clumsy encounter by clapping and hollering throughout Dante's presentations, doing my best to keep busy as hype girl.

Finally, the concealed "Premium Piece" took center stage. This grand finale was a playful gimmick to elicit bids *before* disclosing the art, based on Dante's artist introduction. Alice placed a bulky frame on an easel, facing it backwards towards the crowd. Dante anticipated the artwork, listing accolades of the artist before nodding at me to reveal this cryptic surprise.

Dante started the bid at $15,000, which was my cue to turn the piece towards the crowd. Now, I'm a strong person. Always have been. But there are certain things, like furniture and art frames that require a second pair of hands when repositioning. This thirty-pound, eight-inch-thick mounted hologram by Yaacov Agam was one of such things. I paused in the middle of my pivot, unsure how I would maneuver my body behind the easel without dropping the costly mold of multidimensional lithographs. I caught a frustrated glare from Dante in my peripherals and watched him motion towards Alice to help me. What felt like five minutes later, the two of us successfully propped up the Agam for all to see. I slid off the stage, listening to light applause trickle into silence.

"The bid remains at $15,000... Going once! Going twice!" There were no bids, but Dante's demeanor remained enthusiastic, keeping the audience on their toes.

"And that concludes the auction, ladies and gentlemen. Please be sure to schedule your appointments with one of our lovely associates and ensure a swift checkout for your art in the gallery this evening."

Dante kept his position near the podium to entertain lingering guests commending his performance. Our porters appeared through the "crew only" doors to help break down the set-up of art and easels. Just as I picked up a frame as tall as Charlotte, someone summoned me back towards the stage.

"Jenny!" Dante called out.

I gingerly dropped the artwork in a trolley and gravitated towards his voice.

"For fok sake, man! Quite bliksem, no?!"

Rigid, I sat up like a ventriloquist doll, hoping someone else would speak for me. But alas, the four women remained silent.

Perplexed, I processed Dante's anger and pinned myself as culprit. Unlike my teammates, I did not acquire a bid. However, as a team, we booked an evening of appointments with our biggest leads. So why the rage from Dante? Then, I remembered one of my dad's sentiments: *Some people will never be satisfied.*

We spent the afternoon filing artwork up to the gallery and back into the 'vault,' or a closet of crammed frames. After hanging and dusting and rearranging the art, we had one hour to eat before our first appointment.

I followed Maria and Charlotte to the Lido deck, where we could eat in the guest area before the dinner rush. Alice dipped below deck to visit her boyfriend, a Romanian engineer of whom she had fallen for after starting the job and would eventually marry. Maria then mentioned *her* Romanian boyfriend who worked as a personal trainer on the ship.

"I love him, I do. But I love him as a ship boyfriend." Maria said as she picked at her spread of snacks ranging from waffles to fruit to bagels and lox.

"Watch out Bumblebee, those men will be all over those big eyes of yours. Keep in mind, we get into a relation-*ship*. Your boy becomes just another Facebook friend when your contract ends."

Unimpressed with the handful of crew dudes I had passed on my first day, I shrugged. I was more impressed watching Maria pile up her plate yet remain so thin. I, on the other hand, pretended to enjoy my bowl of fresh cut melon. This contract initiated a fresh start into a mental shift because surely, if I focused on work then my obsession with food would fade away...

"Charlotte, what about you? Do you have a boyfriend?" I asked out of courtesy, considering I deemed her attitude as more business than pleasure.

"Ha" she smirked. "I'm here to work, not to date."

Answer confirmed.

It was nearly 5pm and our first guest would soon visit the gallery for a "free work of art," not including framing and shipping. These "free" works were won from raffles, and those raffles were won by leads.

"Who is Laura Sanders and why is she on the Free Art list?" Dante asked when he strolled in at 4:50pm.

"Oh!" I raised my head from the POS system Charlotte was teaching me to use, set up on a pop-up table for check-outs.

"I spoke to Laura during the auction, and she told me she liked our Robert Wyland mixed media." I answered.

"Is that right?" Dante sneered, unamused.

"Yes, she's a first-time cruiser and stayed throughout the whole auction. I feel good about her." I said.

"It's not about how you *feel*, Jenny. It's whether or not they buy."

I just smiled at him, eager to get back to the POS. *Great advice, Dante. Great advice.*

Guests began filing in and the team advised me to shadow, stay small and silent. Dante and Maria spoke circles around the American guests, charming them with their accents before closing each sale.

Bobbing behind a fine couple dressed for the Captain's Dinner, I caught a glimpse of my fish: Laura Saunders. Her watercolor shawl of cool blues draped over her broad shoulders, allowing the thick rims of her white glasses to really pop. I just hoped those frames would help her to see the beauty of the piece she would soon walk away with.

"Wow! This is Robert Wyland, right?" Laura asked.

"Yes, Laura, it is. The same one we saw this morning." I replied.

"Wasn't there a second one by this artist?" She asked.

"Ah… yes, I'll need to fetch it from the vault. I'll be right back." I said and ran down the corridor.

I slid down the stairs and peeled the art vault open with sweaty hands, frantically searching for the matching piece. *Where in the world was that Wyland?*

After filing through two dozen frames, I caught the whale - Wyland's signature - and ran back up to the sixth deck, stopping a few yards away from the gallery to fan off my face.

"Laura! Here it is!" I lifted the frame just below my chin to watch Laura's reaction.

"Fantastic. I love them." She beamed. Laura was in.

"Yes, fantastic!" I said gleefully. "And lucky for you, we offer a discounted package deal when you buy the same artist. Let's get your shipping information and set you up for the newest addition to your collection!"

Holy hell. I made a sale. For two art works, mind you. I did my best not to do a happy dance in front of Laura, as I was a sales *professional*. And as a professional, closing was a habit along with exuding my cool. We shook hands after Laura signed the invoice for $3,200. Hot damn! I was on fire.

It was 9pm. A potential buyer sat with Dante in deep contemplation over the holographic Agam I had cumbrously revealed earlier at the auction. Dante held the guest's attention with a close grip, then released the older gentleman by assuring him that "this limited edition can only be sold to one guest on this cruise, in which we have plenty of time left on this cruise to decide."

The guest disappeared down the hall just as the art team shuffled into the chapel.

"Mod soka!" Dante shut the doors behind him.

I didn't know what he was yelling in Afrikaans, but it surely wasn't "good job!"

"I can't have you sneaking around like that, Jenny. I can't trust you to close without going through me or Maria first." Dante sniped.

But I made a sale on my first day, what could have possibly gone wrong?

Charlotte stepped in: "Sorry, Dante. I'll work with her to make sure this doesn't happen again."

Disheartened, I sulked in ignorance of my faults, annoyed that I had been spoken for. Dante returned to the gallery's office chair, diving deep into his laptop. I froze, unsure who to seek solace in as Alice looked checked out, Maria furious. I turned to Charlotte and asked, "what did I do?"

She faced me, pausing to collect her patience. "You can't just offer someone a discount, Jenny. If they are willing to pay full price, let them pay full price. You jumped straight to the sale price without asking anyone else to try and upsell your guest. Dante doesn't like that. He wants to have the last say."

Ugh. I wanted a pat on the back, and instead, I was picked apart.

Similar incidents occurred throughout the next month while working for Dante. He did not trust me with the guests, so I did not trust myself with the guests. My sales performance was so-so, and so, I focused on something else I knew I could succeed in: a name for myself below deck.

The Queen Pearl holds around 3,500 guests and 1,200 crew members. Much of this crew came from The Philippines, Indonesia, and India. Throw in a dozen South Africans and Romanians, plus the Italian officers and British dancers. In total, there were five American crew members, including myself, Charlotte, and three Californians working in entertainment. I was young, blonde, and an easy target for attention as the newest addition on board. On my first day, Miguel from Mexico introduced himself as I paced the gallery. He was the maître d for the Cajun steakhouse next door and kissed my hand as he shook it.

"My my, Jennifer from America. Welcome to the Queen Pearl. You are so slim, do you run?"

I nearly choked at the word *slim*. Maria, the petite Romanian, was slim. Alice, the 6'1' South African with the 00 waistline was slim. I scaled at least twenty-five pounds heavier than I did my junior year of college. *That Jenny* was slim. This Jenny had room for improvement, and a reason to run.

"Hi, nice to meet you. Yes, I would call myself a runner." I smiled at Miguel's handsome, tanned face. He had a head full of hair to match his brown eyes. Charming, sure. But a bit too old for my taste, with a flirting approach that was far too pungent.

"How perfect. The crew activities club is throwing a 10k in Skagway next week. The winner for both men and women receive a $500 cash prize, and I don't think there are too many ladies signed up."

Five hundred dollars? Five. Hundred. Dollars. I didn't have one hundred dollars to my name. I could use that cash. And if all else failed, I would get a killer workout.

Without telling my team, I ran as much as possible between shifts to build stamina before the race. I eyed down every female crew member I passed, judging to see who my competition might be before the big day. I guessed the dancers would be my greatest match, given their athletic shape. My curiosity led to inquiry, which led me into the dungy crew bar with three long-legged ladies.

"Hell y'all. Are you in the race?" I asked while sipping a vodka soda. The group looked at one another and giggled.

"Oh honey, I don't run unless I'm being chased." One said.

"I'm running!" Said Erikka, a 19-year-old Australian with a bright smile, perfectly lined in red lipstick.

"Just to get out of rehearsal." Erikka explained.

"What about the cash? Surely, someone in the show has a bigger incentive to run besides missing rehearsal." I probed.

More giggles.

"Bria's going to win. She's our vocalist."

This made sense. Afterall, the vocalists performed two nights out of the seven-day cruise, opening the rest of the week to spend in their leisure. I could be generalizing, but I figured Bria had copious time to run, rest, and repeat before this 10k in Skagway. Whereas I snuck around to train, careful to not tip off Dante. I would run first thing in the morning or late at night as he had us in meetings all day, preventing the art team from visiting our Alaskan ports of call.

"There is nothing to see in Alaska... just bears." He said when I asked about time off at port. But to my surprise, when I asked if I could compete in the race, he sighed, "sure, but you better win."

You got it, boss.

After the guests disembarked in Skagway the next morning, one hundred crew members congregated in the Executive Lounge to obtain their bid numbers for the race. Scanning my competition, I was relieved to see few women racing, and the ones that were did not seem to take the run very seriously. Whereas I kept my focus, queuing up a killer playlist while stretching in my coral pink leggings.

Then I saw her. Bria. She strutted in a matching gray crop top and leggings, showing off her curves and toned muscles from all that time she got to spend at the gym. Potentially the long-lost triplet of Venus and Serena Williams, Bria was tall, beautiful, and fierce. She tied her relaxed hair back, flexing her defined biceps, and swiftly plugged in her earphones to turn on her own pump-up playlist. I sensed her gaze drop towards my pink leggings, wondering who this white girl was signing up for the race so late in the game.

The runners clustered through the security gates and made their way towards the starting line half a mile from shore. I stepped off the ship for the first time in four days, liberating my lungs with fresh Alaskan air. A vast landscape of white mountains bordered the tiny town of red, blue, yellow, and orange buildings. As the dock's runway dropped us off on the streets of Skagway, we migrated onto the set of a Western film. The showdown was about to begin.

Alongside me were four dancers, all wearing bright sportswear and flawless makeup. Their insouciant banter was fun until I saw the announcer's block, where I excused myself to focus.

"I'll wait for you at the finish line, guys. I gotta win this race." I said as I broke off from their casual pace and squeezed my way through the crowd.

"BANG"

Shots fired.

"Go Jenny!" shouted the dance crew behind me. Then I heard another voice from the spectators.

"Ya Jenny!"

To my surprise, it was Charlotte, standing in a black windbreaker and baseball cap. I did not ask or expect anyone from the gallery to show up for me, but here she was, on my team, *rooting* for me. This sense of patriotism helped me conjure up more strength to win the cash prize.

Unfortunately, patriotism does not protect you from altitude and incline. The race started entirely uphill, a path consisting of lightly beaten switchbacks and narrow trails parting a sea of birch trees. I watched my footing to avoid slipping on mud, though fallen spruce covered the trail and provided traction. Most participants tapered off after ten minutes, though I had yet to pass Bria. By the third mile I was running alone in the Alaskan rainforest, enchanted by a veil of green, intoxicated by the cool mist. Bright lime moss draped the forest floor, releasing an invigorating scent of pine and morning dew. At the end of the grove, the route rounded out towards a paved road descending down the mountain. I knew that once the incline was over, it was literally downhill from here.

The skyline cleared out to a snow tipped mountain range separated by the crystal waters of the Skagway River. That's when I saw her. Bria. She treaded slowly, losing speed. Watching her pace, I reminded myself that I was a swimmer at heart, and a miler at that. Distance is my forte. Stamina is my strength. I revved up my internal engine and finished this endurance race.

I shot Bria a wave as I passed her, leaving her in shock. As the road curved down the rocky mountain, colliding colors of the town's infrastructure pierced through a horizon of natural hues. With two miles to go and five hundred dollars to win, I *sprinted* that last leg as if I was chased by an Alaskan grizzly. I showed no mercy. The spiraling path led me back into town, where crew members cheering on the sidewalks yelled, "You've got this! She's not even close."

But how could I judge? Sweat stung my eyes. The runner's high warped reality. I could sense that Bria gave up after I cruised past her, picking up speed. Though I couldn't count on it. I could only count on myself.

The pavement leveled out. I peered through perspiration, making out a figure in the distance - Miguel from Mexico stood on a platform, throwing up a high-five to someone in celebration. To my right, Charlotte cheered behind a galvanized barrier in delight. Counting footsteps, I reached sixty-two until the finish line was soon behind me. Legs shaking, I bent over to catch my knees and coughed up saliva. No need to hold back tears, coughs, or cries. Appearance was the last thing on my mind. Because despite my sweaty, disheveled state, I had established higher echelon on board and my reputation would precede my next appearance.

Half an hour later, I stood on top of the awards podium to receive my first-place medal, my cash prize, and a bottle of Veuve Clicquot Champagne. I wobbled back onto the Queen Pearl with my bubbly and an enhanced sense of bravado, just in time to shower before 'Pick the Price.'

An air of arrogance clung to my clothes as I sauntered into the gallery. To my surprise, my team greeted me with praise.

"Bumblebee! I can't believe you did it! I didn't think you could win!" said Maria in all earnestness.

"Ah. It's the pink bear!" boasted Dante.

"Come again?" I asked.

"I went out to ship a package this morning and saw something pink dash past me and could have sworn it was a bear. But it was your bright bottoms... Anyways, good job, bear."

"Thank you, Dante!"

My word! Dante acknowledged me *and* gave me a nickname.

"Girls, you can wrap up 'Pick the Price' at 8pm tonight. I've made a reservation at the steakhouse to celebrate another win for the art team. Dinner is on me, but the champagne is on Jenny."

I finally allowed myself to relax around my coworkers that evening, which was easy considering how fast the champagne hit after the alpine run. On Dante's dime, I indulged in fried oysters, seasoned hushpuppies, seafood gumbo and a butterflied beef filet. I did not save room for my buttermilk bread pudding, but I ate it anyway, licking up every inch of the pistachio caramel sauce with delight. I allowed this gluttonous behavior to endure after weeks of anxiously restricting from sales training and onboarding, justifying the number of calories I had burned from the race. But the hunger didn't halt after the bread pudding. The gorging had only begun.

Unfortunately, Dante's fury returned the next night during an exclusive event for previous art collectors. Expecting a high-profile attendance, we displayed our finest works and served complimentary brut and hors d'oeuvres... It didn't pay off.

"Fok all!" Dante flicked a plastic flute off a table, firing sparks of brut into the air.

"I can't be carrying your weight all cruise." He continued.

"Get to your cabins and figure out how we can make some god damned money tomorrow."

Maria, Charlotte, and Alice quietly dispersed. I tiptoed after them until -

"Jenny!" Dante barked.

What did I do this time?

"Stay in the gallery until ten in case anyone comes through." Dante said as he strolled out, fuming.

There I was, alone with artwork that cost as much as my college tuition and a leftover plate of cheese.

I wrapped up at exactly ten, sharper than the cubes of cheddar. My tummy moaned as I moped towards my cabin. Aggravated, I knew I wasn't the strongest on the team, but that didn't make me weak.

You are ok, Jenny. You haven't even been working for a month. You still have time to shine.

My inner cheerleader pepped me up before another voice started to impede.

Fuck it. Fuck this. Dante doesn't care about you. He cares about money. So why should <u>you</u> care about you?

Somehow, I found myself in the crew cafeteria. An aroma of curried chicken filled the room along with the dozens of male house workers speaking Bengali, Hindi and Filipino. Heads lifted at every table I walked by, flashing toothy grins at the only woman in the room.

With everyone watching, I avoided eye contact and made ways towards the food. I had eaten more than enough gouda and dried apricots at the event, but that wasn't enough. I ate grapes and rosemary crackers, too, but still, I didn't feel complete. With all eyes on me in this crammed cafeteria, I began piling up my plate, hoping the voyeurs would cast their gaze away from such a deplorable sight. Starting with a tray of petit fours, I found a corner to eat in solitude. The cakes softened easily on my tongue, disappearing just as I stood up to go back in line. In this round, I recruited chocolate eclairs into a red, opaque drinking glass and took the cup to the soft serve machine. Tongue swelling, I watched the ice cream press through the metal mouth.

Jenny! Stop! What are you doing?

Thoughts started racing… no, *screaming* so loud, I worried I'd disturb the Indonesian man waiting in line behind me.

Jesus, Jenny! You must have eaten 4,000 calories today! And tomorrow is auction day! When do you expect to exercise and undo this damage?

"Hush!" I said to the noise. "I'll figure out a way."

I returned to my seat and scooped up my mixture, slowly dipping my spoon to make the flavor last. But during a binge, nothing ever lasts long.

I told myself: *just one more thing, then please walk away.* Grabbing two boxes of Apple Jacks, I reasoned that the cereal counted as one item. I poured the sugary circles into a bowl, added milk, and dug in.

After the final scoop, I stared at my plate of crumbs, my dirty plastic cup, and the last drops of 2% still left in my bowl. I had hollowed out the dishes, stuffing myself with dread. Before dispensing my tray into the dish pit, I slid the spoon from my cereal into my blazer's pocket. Four thousand calories were not about to weigh me down. Exercise was out of the question for the next 24 hours. Running out of options, I scurried up to the sixth deck to a space I knew no guest would roam at this time of night. Ten yards down from the gallery, an open, single stall bathroom awaited me.

The cycle of stress-induced binging and purging progressed over the next month. While I was building rapport with my teammates, steadily selling more art, and drinking dollar beers with the dancers most nights, I regretted how much I had to be "on." And because Charlotte and I shared the same schedule, I was rarely alone in my cabin, provoking a restlessness that sent me out to scour the ship for food.

When Dante delivered my 30-day evaluation, he told me I was "an attractive woman, which can be a great advantage in sales", but I "needed to know where I stand" and that I was "too impulsive", all while telling me this "from a professional perspective".

Truthfully, I did not take offense from this evaluation, nor did I catch creepy vibes from Dante's comment on my appearance. But I was uncomfortable. I summarized the report as: "at least you don't suck!" calculating all the ways I could improve.

One sunny day in Ketchikan, Dante called the art team together for an impromptu meeting. He waited for us in the gallery, wearing a childish grin.

"I'm being transferred to the Celestial Seas in Barcelona."

The girls all gasped.

"Starting next cruise... Your new auctioneers are a Canadian couple. I've never heard of either of them, but they've been in the business since the late 90's. Best of luck."

Thrilled, the room took a collective sigh. Canadians were notoriously *nice*. And best of all, they were not Dante.

After my first two months, the art team shifted significantly. Alice left for vacation to plan her wedding with the Romanian engineer. Charlotte transferred to Hawaii, and I moved into a larger cabin with Maria.

Meanwhile, my curly haired associates were replaced by Gabriel and Mika, a playful, petite couple from Romania. While the pair was quick to crack jokes, they were serious in closing a sale. Gabriel and Mika consented with constructive feedback, all with patience and care. After a turbulent first stretch of my contract, cruise life would be smooth sailing from here.

My new auctioneers, Paul and Michelle, embarked on the Queen Pearl just as the ship headed south to reposition to Fort Lauderdale. During this 18-day cruise, we would sail for two weeks down California and Mexico, cut through the locks of the Panama Canal, and reach the Caribbean ports of

Aruba, Jamaica, Grand Cayman, and Costa Rica. The day before this grand departure, Michelle messaged the team on Facebook to let us know the Canadian couple would greet everyone at muster drill.

With their life vests in hand, I immediately recognized them. The two strutted down the runway with million-dollar smiles. Paul's fading brown hair was still perfectly intact and gelled back, framing his tanned face which floated above his sharp gray suit and purple bow tie.

Then there was Michelle. Mature and elegant, she exuded youth. Her smile spread as wide as Julia Roberts, with an energy just as warm and welcoming.

"Hey team!" Paul reached his hand out for all to shake, instantly resetting the tone from the gallery's former auctioneer. His vibe was gregarious and goofy, carrying an arsenal of experience and tacky dad jokes. His girlfriend Michelle was by his side to nervously laugh at said jokes, adding a side of eye roll. From day one, I sensed I could trust my new auctioneers, and that this mutual respect would exceed my best sales day while working with Dante.

Where Dante discouraged exercise, Paul and Michelle did so daily, embodying everything I would want to be at their age. Shortly after joining the Queen Pearl, our auctioneers simultaneously celebrated their fortieth and forty-first birthday and invited the team out for drinks. Though before we said "cheers," Michelle insisted we meet in the gallery for cake where there was ample lighting to unveil Paul's gift for her big 4-0.

"O my god," Maria held me back with her hand, saving me from emotional whiplash.

"Paul! You didn't!" Maria yelled.

"He sure did." beamed Michelle.

Michelle looked stunning as always, allowing her cropped black trousers to effortlessly outline her Barbie-thin legs.

Michelle took a spin, revealing a red leather bottom to her jet-black shoes.

"They're beautiful," pleaded Maria.

Paul had surprised Michelle with a pair of classic Christian Louboutin's, after hearing her drip subtle references around her affinity for the iconic pump. While these shoes cost more than the amount in my bank account, I felt fancy by association.

Michelle posted a photo of her present on Facebook, accruing over 200 likes in her red bottoms. During this time, I was also gaining traction on my social media game. Friends commented on my photos from the ports, responding with "You're so lucky" and "Do you just travel?" Though after the initial ping of dopamine dissipated, I wasn't so sure if I felt "liked'" as much as I did "seen." But no one saw me laboring over 16-hour days. And while I portrayed a luxury lifestyle of nomadic exploration, those wanderlust posts were a mere filter to cover up how lost I truly was.

...

While I admired her body, I never envied Michelle. Her smile faded when she thought no one was watching, but I caught her indifference towards ship life and that she was ready to return home. Michelle only spoke with kindness, something I tried to embody as much as I tried to mirror her self-control to eat well and exercise. Over the weeks, Michelle's diligence slightly rubbed off on me, yet the void inside persisted. I continued to stuff this void in silence and isolation. And while my binging decreased slightly after Dante transferred, a wickedness within remained:

Michelle is a size 2, and she's forty. Why can't you follow suit? Why can't you just go back to seventeen where you could scan a table full of food without making a move? How are buffets on the ship any different than your college cafeteria? Why can't you control your intake like you did then? Where'd that girl go? Where's your god-damned will power?

I started implementing fruit-only days and intermittent fasting. This of course backfired into a spiral of ravenous eating parades. I started to sneak into various buffets, sure to eat a suitable amount at each deck so no one would catch the attractive, athletic, art associate stuffing her face, plate after plate.

Work was not enough to keep me from binging—it hardly slowed me down. In the amount of time one would excuse themselves to the restroom, I'd sneak out of an auction, race down to the crew mess and snatch up sweets served during "happy hour." I'd pocket a trio of chocolate chip cookies into a napkin, eat the first one on the walk back towards the guest area, shove in the second one behind the door leading into the guest area, and nibble on the third throughout the auction, pretending to cough as I licked chocolate off my lips.

Grease started to stain my clothes. My fingernails were always filthy, and a breakout on my chin was evidence of a sugar overdose. The previous year when preparing to study abroad, I was eating more carbs in proper proportions. My parents told me I looked "strong and healthy," and I believed them. More importantly - I saw myself in this way. But somewhere during my Italian escapades, I took the traveling advice, "say yes to everything" a little too literally. I said yes - and could not stop. Years of restricting calories were catching up with me. I had starved myself for so long that my hunger was now rebounding in revenge. I was no longer controlling my food. The food was controlling me.

...

One night after a big sale, Maria insisted she take the team out to a preset dinner at the Italian restaurant next to the gallery. Thrilled to take her offer on an expensed indulgence, I said, "sì" with enthusiasm. Paul and Michelle, however, politely refused.

"Thanks Maria, but we already had our cheat meal of the week. Gotta watch the figure in both body *and* business, you know?" Paul was selling Maria on his excuse, but I wasn't buying any of it.

I was flooded with judgment, thinking how selfish our auctioneers were to honor their health over socializing. But this judgment was a mere reflection of myself, angry that I would jump at any opportunity to eat. Even if it meant sabotaging my team.

After the Italian dinner, which, of course was delectable as any meal coated with fat, oil and salt would be, Maria headed to her boyfriend's cabin. I went back to ours to play solitaire. When Maria got "home," she took a cigarette to the bathroom where she smoked through the vent. I panicked.

"Hola Bumblebee" Maria came out immediately, before sparking up.

"Jenny. Are you throwing up?" She asked straightforwardly.

Unsure of what to say and how she knew, the evidential smell started to leak out the bathroom door.

"Jenny, I had a cabinmate who used to throw up, and she was not well. You don't have to do that, dear. Just don't eat as much, ok?" Maria said solemnly.

"Just don't eat as much… OK?"

OK? No, not ok. Please, Maria, teach me how you do it. Tell me how you fill your plate with delectable treats then, quite wastefully, eat only half of what you take. Tell me how you fit into a size 0 without working out. And please, please tell me that my capricious cravings can be calmed by simply… *not eating as much.*

"Yes, sorry Maria. I felt so sick after all that pasta. I promise it won't happen again." I responded quietly.

Maria believed me, and for a moment, I had us both fooled. My shame lasted long enough to prevent another binge that week, though time was no remedy for my untreated insanity. My logic was that if Maria never *caught* me throwing up again, I would keep my promise.

"Bumblebee! Do you know what day it is?" She raved.

"It's the first day of your last cruise before vacation." I affirmed.

"Yes." She beamed. "Yes, it is."

I was happy for Maria to take leave, I truly was. But I was not ready for the art team to make another one-eighty. The three Romanians were heading home just in time for Christmas, whereas the auctioneers and I still had eight weeks to complete our contract. Eighteen weeks had passed since stepping onto the Queen Pearl, tallying 126 days since having any "time off." As when you work on ships, you're always *on*, and I was experiencing major burn out. Fortunately, Paul and Michelle encouraged me to see the ports when we docked. Thus, I made it my job to paddle board along the placid beaches in Aruba and snorkel off the coast of the Grand Cayman Islands, documenting with my GoPro, posting it all on my budding Instagram. And despite being a swimmer by nature, no amount of watersports could provide the same familiarity of home, weekends, couches, groceries and of other land-locked nuances we take for granted when living below sea level. Still, I swam in the ocean every chance I could get, reminding myself that I chose this career, and that was a great privilege.

While docked one December morning in Ft. Lauderdale, I met Maria, Gabriel, and Mika in the crew bar where they would receive their detained passports for disembarkation. For the first time, I saw Maria cry. I cried. We all cried and said our final goodbyes. I had found a family among strangers, and in a matter of minutes, I would never see any of them again. Desolate, I remembered when Maria had warned me from my first day that everything ends the moment your contract does. That all the people you bond with for that intense amount of time will return home to a distant land. We may continue to "like" each other via social media, but everyone you meet in this world of cruising ends up being a short-lived relation-*ship.*

...

My next all-star team consisted of Omar, an Egyptian gallery director; Starr, my newest South African roommate; and Nick from New Jersey, an art associate who was brand-spanking new to ships. Paul was ecstatic to have Omar as he had worked with some of the top producing auctioneers in the company and arrived packing high-performing evaluations from his latest assignment. Omar's chocolate skin wrapped tightly around his bones. He kept his black hair buzzed and wore metal frames that outlined his solemn, pensive stare. While not as organized as Maria – though who could blame him, he was new – Omar's direct communication style whipped me into shape by being hyper involved, adding constructive insight each time he observed me speaking to guests. And while he scared the shit out of me and insisted I close *every* sale, he worked closely with me so we could all succeed. There were aspects of Omar's approach that reminded me of Dante, however Omar's tactics were based on teamwork and technique, rather than control.

Starr was two years my senior with tanned skin, wild brown curls, and a refreshing, laid back attitude. She had worked on ships for a few years now, eager to be reunited with her Romanian boyfriend as requested in her contract. This got me wondering, should *I* be pursuing a Romanian boyfriend? They surely were sprinkled around ships like candy, though most of their rough demeanors weren't sweet enough for me to chew.

Then there was Nick. Sweet, little Nick. Little in how he spoke and took up space, despite being lengthy, blonde, and bony. Nick came on board aloof and a little lost, but hey, who was I to judge considering my main motive for working on ships was to chase likes online. But by the time Nick started his contract, I was starting to invest myself fully into this job. After being a little hard on him one day, I invited him for a drink in the crew bar to apologize and show him my "fun" side.

"Cheers, man. Sorry I've been rough on you lately. I just want us all to thrive. From what I've learned, the contract goes by a lot smoother when we're hitting numbers. But I'm curious, why'd you apply for this job?" I asked Nick after small talk and a couple brews.

"Honestly?" Nick hesitated.

"Yea, honestly… it's better than bullshit." I teased.

"I was told there's a lot of Asians on board. I'm looking for a ladyboy." He replied.

"Oh. Good for you." It certainly wasn't what I expected, but it wasn't bullshit, either.

It seemed as if everyone had a specific agenda for their time on board, and all I had was a corner in the crew cafeteria. Eventually, my loneliness led me to a place where loneliness was welcomed, all for a low, low cost. I now regularly stepped into the crew bar to order a Blue Moon for a dollar, before men from photog spent a few more dollars for me. Such generosity was granted after befriending the photography team on the Promenade deck, as they sold portraits next to the gallery's "Pick the Price" table.

When it comes to romance, I believe in the following three levels of attraction: love-at-first-sight, liquor-induced, or a slow-burn infatuation. According to the psychology of attraction, two major components of allurement are proximity and frequency. Meaning when you eat, drink, and work alongside someone within a six-month contract, some kind of coital conduct is sure to ensue.

Frederich the photog was from Cape Town, South Africa and just a year older than me. While I didn't think twice about my first sighting of Frederich, a slow burn of cordial conversations led to a sloppy string of flings. One night in crew bar, silver PVC streamers lined the dancefloor for a disco party. I bopped by head to funky beats, barely seeing out the pair of inordinate pink sunglasses I found sprinkled about the bar. Donna Summer's "Last Dance" came on to signal the last call, which prompted Frederich to offer to walk me back to my cabin. Cute, Frederich, real cute. Because on land, a guy friend offering a gal pal a ride or walk home *can* show genuine concern for her safety. Below deck, this good deed implies one thing. Frederich led me down the brightly lit, surveilled hallway and into my dark, empty room. The deed was about to be done.

Two pow-wows later, I found myself hugging onto the toilet for dear mercy. It wasn't a purge, but an abominable UTI. Unable to work, I confronted Michelle to inform her what was going on and she dismissed me from the gallery with stern, sisterly advice to stay safe below deck. When released, I chugged cranberry juice between painful pees then vomited up the excess liquids I tried forcing down to stay hydrated. Vacillating between toilet to bed, bed to floor, and back to the porcelain throne that had me chained, I was a mad, sad, infected harbor of flesh.

I soon showed up to the medical center a hot, sweaty mess. The doctor opened the clinic, shocked to see me. And while he could have been thrown off by my ruffled appearance, we were both startled to see each other again since sleeping together just a week prior.

Elijah, a South African doctor, and I fondled one another after a night of heavy imbibing at crew bar. But given our drastically different schedules and work locations, I hardly ever passed him on the ship. This second meet-cute was anything but after I gave him a sample of my urine to determine that it was in fact infected.

"I'm administering phenazopyridine and three days of antibiotics. If the pain doesn't subside after that, come back to see me." Elijah advised.

I nodded, eager to jet and let the meds do their magic. Before leaving, Elijiah added:

"Oh, and be sure to release your bladder after any sexual activity."

...

The drugs turned my pee orange and alleviated pressure off my lower organs. This boost gave me the strength to awkwardly explain to Frederich why we couldn't have sex for a few days.

"You have a *UTI?!*" he echoed.

"Yes, do you know what a UTI is, Frederich?" I felt like his mother. Not exactly a turn on.

"Uh..." He mumbled.

"So, a U-T-I is a urinary tract infection. It's common among women, though it can happen to men. But don't worry. They're not contagious." I explained.

Once I finished my 3-day pack of antibiotics, I found myself back at the crew bar. Because Frederich and I had already been friends before we exchanged benefits, no one suspected any recent breakthroughs out of the friend zone. Besides, I acted purely platonic towards Frederich in public. So, when Elijah sat down next to me as I was sitting next to Frederich, neither man knew what the hell was going on.

For the next half hour, I was sandwiched between two lovers, thanking God that the lights were dim enough to hide my profuse perspiration. At one point, I swear both men had their hand on my shoulder, clueless to each other's advances. To avoid a messy conversation, I excused myself after one beer that night and headed back to my cabin alone.

I was at a crossroads. I had developed a friendship with Frederich, which allowed me to soften my inhibitions around him. This rose-colored filter was a case of "ship eyes," a phenomenon more colloquially known as "camp eyes," meaning when you're stuck at camp with a limited group of individuals for an extended amount of time, you'll eventually fall for *someone*.

Now, I found Elijah attractive, but we barely had a relationship outside my visits to the crew bar and the health clinic, of which neither were particularly sexy. At the same time, I felt indebted to Frederich because I had led him on for the past week and we would both take vacation in a matter of four. What was worse, I felt Frederich falling for me, and I intended to stand my ground by staying single. The problem was, I didn't have the heart to tell him.

The closer Frederich and I inched towards vacation, the tighter our bond fastened. He started dropping love notes in my cabin's key slot, and I left him KitKats by the photo stands with a Post-it reading, "I hope you catch a break today <3". We drank at crew bar every night and stayed up late to watch Rick and Morty. On the rarity we both had down time to spend at port together, we would. One day in Jamaica, we did.

"Mary-wanna?" A tall Jamaican man in a Bob Marley tee whispered to me and Frederich as we walked down the commercial strip in Ocho Rios. We looked at each other and giggled, bought the grass and papers, and found a bench in an inconspicuous park to roll a joint. With a doobie in hand, we headed to Mystic Mountain, a scenic ski-lift attraction that takes you up a lush rainforest and back down for a panoramic view of the aquamarine Caribbean Sea. We bought a Sky Explorer ticket and lit up the joint as our seat lifted us over the Jamaican jungle. Getting stoned with my sweetheart helped me escape from the stress of art sales, though the come down left me wondering what would remain of this relation-ship once our contracts ended.

Later, after a 'Pick-The-Price' shift, crew drinks, and contraband tokes through the bathroom vent, Frederich and I were alone in his cabin. We mentioned vacation and our impending separation. I told him I wanted to visit him in South Africa, which was true. And I also told him I loved him, which was very much drug induced.

He didn't reciprocate that night, and I never said those words again. Because while I loved Frederich for his friendship, his softness, and the kindness he spread, I was never *in* love with him. And that one little preposition makes all the difference.

The next day, Frederich and I sat down to discuss my now imminent trip to Cape Town. Booking my flight implied commitment past our contracts, which brought up Frederich's aspirations to apply for a position with Galleries at Sea. This also brought up what I had said the night before, those three burning words.

"Jenny, we were drunk and high last night. I don't know if you remember what you said, but I want you to know I feel the same way. But I also can't tell if you said it *because* you were drunk and high, so you don't have to feel like you have to say it again unless you really mean it." As these heavy words left his lips, his deep brown eyes stayed light and locked on mine.

While Frederich displayed an immense amount of vulnerability that morning, I had lost the liquid courage from the night before to express how I felt. I smiled at him in silence for a moment, and replied, "They say alcohol reveals the truth. And the truth is, I'm not ready to say what I said last night again. But I care for you, deeply, and I am grateful for this relationship. Whatever happens to us after vacation, know that you'll always be my special friend."

Frederich swallowed at that last word: *friend.* Though for at least one more month, this friendship would prove itself beneficial. I then clicked "book" for my flight to Cape Town, extending the expiration date of our personal contract a wee bit longer, knowing very well that when that trip would end, so would this accord.

After six months of living underwater, I had worked under two sets of auctioneers, two different gallery directors, and alongside six different art associates. Starting in Vancouver, B.C., I had won a 10k race in Skagway and ate crab legs as big as my forearm in Juneau, Alaska. I set foot in South America for the first time during our reposition cruise to Fort Lauderdale, ready to spend the winter in the Caribbean. Once the Queen Pearl sailed through warmer waters, I paddle boarded off immaculate beaches. I swam with stingrays. I hiked up waterfalls. I zip-lined through Costa Rican jungles and I smoked pot in Jamaica. I made lovers out of men from around the world. But as I portrayed this glamorous lifestyle on my Instagram feed, I lost so much of myself.

I was "living my best life" and posting the highlights on social media. And yet, I still wasn't fulfilled. While I slept below deck, everything felt surface level. The art I sold started to seem fabricated, as "limited edition" works were just copies. Near the end, the fading smiles of my fellow crew members began to feel fake. We were all here to put on a show for paying guests, then cash out and leave. With crew members taking vacation and transferring ships each week, veterans advised against any scale of emotional attachment. And that came from Maria, a woman I considered family when we worked together. But by the time I departed the Queen Pearl in January of 2015, I was ready for reunions with those whose lives seemed a lot more stable than mine at sea.

During my month-long vacation, I spent every weekend in a new city, couch surfing with old friends as they embraced me with open arms.

"It's the world traveler!" High school, college and former colleague friends would say each time I stepped foot inside a familiar, land-locked bar. Soon, that title had become synonymous with my name, as I had picked up a bit of notoriety during my six months at sea. Every night I went out, an old acquaintance would approach me and admit that they had been following my social media.

"I just love what you're doing, Jenny. I live my life vicariously through your Instagram."

I'm sorry, what was your name?

Surely, I was flattered. And I loved that I could inspire others with travel, never mind expose them to parts of the world they would have never thought to explore. But when the drinks wore off in the morning, these comments left me repulsed.

Did I dare tell them what was really going on? Should I have brushed off their compliments and said, "yea, well, don't get *too* vicarious. I'm bulimic." Of course not, because at the dawn of 2015, I wasn't bulimic—not in my mind. I was just someone who thought about my body, food, and exercise 90% of my day. Besides, I was binging and purging *only* once a week. I had a problem, yes. But I had goals. I had a unique career which allowed me to pursue those goals. And I wasn't going to let a little disease get in my way.

I visited Frederich at the tail-end of my vacation, spending seven days with him in a suburb outside of Cape Town. His parents welcomed me with wide, heavy hugs and his younger brother adored my playful, American attitude. I was treated like a princess, but I surely didn't feel like one.

One morning, Frederich and I hiked Lion's Head to catch breathless views of Table Mountain, an extrusive landmark that surrounds the city. It was particularly windy that morning as we traversed the three-mile incline. Dirt from the trail billowed up into dust and our hoods tugged at our necks. Frederich continuously asked if I was doing ok, which bothered me. At the summit, where a horizon of royal blue waters crashed along the rocky coast, Frederich reached out his hand to help lift me to higher ground.

"I'm fine." I brushed his hand away and pushed myself up a boulder. The city skyline appeared from the vantage point, vast and majestic and protected by the surrounding mountains. Frederich and I watched over his city in silence. Once when we made our way back to his car, Frederich broke our quiet descent. "You really don't like to be helped, do you?"

That afternoon, we drove through rolling hills painted in a hundred hues of green to spend a romantic night in the coastal town of Hermanus. It would be our only night sleeping in the same bed, as his parents put me up in a guest room back in the suburbs. Our suite faced the rocky beaches and rough, dark waters, where we spent our last moments of intimacy. Before the sun rose the next morning, we drove another hour to Gansbaai to suit up and cage dive with great-white sharks. Taking a small tugboat a couple kilometers offshore, dozens of seagulls circled around us as the captain threw fish chum into the sea. The sharks didn't scare me as much as the biting temperature of the water. Besides, these excursions ran 365 days a year, taking tourists from around the world into the Indian Ocean. It seemed that the sharks got the best deal out of this gig, with free breakfast every morning. However, I was undercaffeinated, cold and caged.

Frederich and I left no day unattended, maxing out each hour to sightsee. We drank wine throughout the college campus of Stellenbosch and watched penguins flock around the sandy boulders of Simon's Beach. We made love when we could, and eventually, we had a conversation about the future of this atypical relationship.

Frederich wanted to work for the art gallery, and he wanted to work with me. This would mean adjoining a contract together, splitting paychecks and cabins for a six-month stint. The thought alone shot intense pressure into my chest. This instinct told me that I wasn't ready for a relationship, nor was I willing to share my career with someone I had only known in a circumstantial environment. Frederich understood, though he longed for a different response. I wished him the best of luck and promised we would stay in touch.

Frederich waited by the gate at the Cape Town International airport until I faded away through security. He was one of the first people to greet me during my six-month contract on the Queen Pearl, and one of the last to say goodbye before I headed back to Miami for another sales training. We were never meant to be, but we remained friends. There was no heartbreak when the romance died down, only gratitude for a man who held me for a blink of time - a time of which everything felt as fluid as the waters we lived upon.

My month-long vacation left me refreshed and ready to show up for round two of training. From my travels across America to an incredible week in South Africa, I was determined to keep the momentum alive. My hunger for success drove me to ask for a promotion to gallery director, and what you ask for, my friends, you shall receive.

...

Bringing a refreshed spirit and a smidge of arrogance into training, I was feeling *real* hot in Miami. So hot, that I requested a promotion *within* my next contract, considering how competent I felt when leaving the Queen Pearl. To my surprise, Galleries at Sea threw me into the deep end of an entirely new shark tank, with no cage to save me this time.

I stepped into my new assignment as gallery director for the Bella Fiesta, a ship positioned out of Port Canaveral, Florida with a route around the Eastern Caribbean. My auctioneer was Lewis, a short Irish man with a hairstyle so suave, it added a couple inches to his overall height. Lewis partnered with his girlfriend, Molly, who was a year older than me and a fellow Midwesterner. Despite our similarities, however, Molly had a cunning vibe behind her round blue eyes and porcelain teeth. After a curt introduction with Lewis and Molly, I was already missing my Canadian couple, Paul and Michelle.

The art associates were less than enthused to greet their young, American gallery director step into their space with a skirt and ponytail. Within minutes of cringy banter, I soon learned that Gerrie from South Africa hardly hid his racism from our Black Zimbabwean colleague, Tawana. And once Gerrie had a couple drinks in him, which was any time he wasn't in the gallery, his misogyny wreaked wildly through the help of his pal, Jim Beam.

As gallery director, it was now my responsibility to help administer the team and close the big leads. But selling seemed insurmountable as I spent my energy suppressing flippant remarks from my coworkers, which cut through the core of my deepest wounds.

To ease those wounds, I ate. And ate, and ate, and ate. My eating spiraled as I pinballed around the ship, darting from a burger buffet to the soft serve ice cream machine. At night, I waited patiently for my cabinmate to head to the crew bar before I snuck up to the Lido deck for slices from the 24-hour pizza parlor. I then tried drinking cheap white wine with melatonin after work in hopes of passing out before I could binge. I contemplated cigarettes, but that would require me to smoke in designated areas, which seemed too social for the loneliness I was trying to subdue on my own.

When my birthday arrived in late June, 24-year-old Molly told me that "23 was the worst year of her life." Before she told me this, I had already learned from Blink-182 that no one likes you when you're 23, and I was about to experience this aversion firsthand.

The night of my birthday, the art team and I closed out the crew bar as Lewis and Gerrie kept buying rounds of tequila shots. After five, maybe six rounds, I was the first to tap out. I snuck up to the Lido deck for pizza and spent the rest of my night vomiting up the alcohol. The next day, Tawana confessed that Lewis and Gerrie were only buying tequila for me, while the rest of the team drank water when we cheered.

This news made me sick again, and it wasn't from the tequila. I was humiliated, I felt betrayed. I kept eating to fill this pain, which made the hurt exacerbate.

Like any substance, there is a difference and a spectrum between a normie (eater) and (a food) addict. Normal eaters overeat from time to time, and addicts, well, it's much more complicated than that. I have a hunch that every human living in a developed country has eaten past full at least once in their life. I've witnessed it everywhere. In person. On TV. I've seen a normal eater polish off a plate, rub their belly, refer to their food baby, even joke about "going anorexic" for the next week, then carry on with their night and go back to their normal eating habits the next day. What shocks me isn't when people humor disordered eating as a remedy, but that they can go back to their normal eating habits after indulging. I, on the other hand, would just be getting started.

This illuminates the difference between a person who has overeaten and a food addict. A food addict cannot stop. As much as their abdomen pains them to put down their fork, the connection between the brain and their feverish hand is lost. A food addict stops caring about weight, about image and about the repercussions during a binge. The addictive mind starts screaming:

FOOD. FAT. SO FAT. MORE FOOD. MORE. MORE. NOT ENOUGH. NOT ENOUGH FOOD. THIS WILL NEVER BE ENOUGH FOOD. FOOD. FAT. YOU ARE FAT. YOU ARE SO FUGLY AND FAT. YOU ARE NOT ENOUGH.

Such thoughts raced through my head as I purged in my cabin shortly after my birthday "celebration." I coughed up all sorts of carbs in my stall whilst my cabinmate was away at work. This cabinmate was a houseworker from Thailand, as human resources had matched new onboards to live with me until they could coordinate rooms for them to live with another employee in the same position. It was now my fourth month on the Bella Fiesta, and I was on my fourth cabinmate. HR had matched me with a Thai housekeeper, a Peruvian housekeeper, and once with a Jamaican housekeeper who had never worked on ships before. This woman wept each night for the children she left back at home. Once a week, the Bella Fiesta would dock in Port Canaveral and my revolving cabin door would swap out a new soul to embark on a grossly long contract away from their country and loved ones. I would listen as these housekeepers called their families, and while I was unable to translate their language, I could still hear their pain. I felt their exhaustion as they returned from a long day of work, after monotonous duties and thankless chores. These women chose ships to generate American currency to send back to their families, whereas I chose ships for the free rent and travel. My multiple roommates and I led drastically different lives, but we all shared the same sorrow of missing home.

I tried to stay grateful. For the opportunity, for the experience. I tried to see the beauty in my time at sea, capturing it all on my Instagram. I anticipated likes, and I rode them out until the hunger for acceptance returned between posts. But each time I read the comment "I want your life," I hated myself more.

Why? Why would you want to be me? Can't you see? You may dread your cubicle back home in America, but I am trapped on a boat with my head in a toilet.

There I was, newly twenty-three and down on my knees. I stared into the metal bin of shame, pressing the lever to make it go away.

Flush

Nothing.

I pulled the lever once more, but my regurgitated meals remained.

NO!

Hunched over with one hand on toilet seat and the other gripping the end of a toothbrush, I waited another minute before trying to drown out what I had just done.

Nothing.

SHIT!

Memories of my onboard training flashed as violently as the vomit I had just forced up my esophagus. We were warned as crew members to not flush feminine products and large wads of toilet paper down the latrine, as the ship's pipes are much smaller than those on land. My breath became shorter. My heart was starting to sting. What would happen if I had clogged the toilet indefinitely? If I broke the flow of the ship's septic system? The guest's toilets were surely starting to overfill, the kitchen sinks must have come to a cease. The onboard engineers would track the fault back to me. Everyone would find out what I had done.

I couldn't breathe. I couldn't think. No, I couldn't *stop thinking*. I hopped out of the bathroom and unnervingly looked into the full-length mirror.

WHAT HAVE YOU DONE?

I asked the monster in my reflection to go away and ripped off my clothes to lighten the load of remorse trapped on my skin. Grabbing onto the ladder to my top bunk, I shook it steadily as I eased up to my bed. Still shaking, I slipped under my sheets, curled into a ball, and cried into my pillow. I wanted to suffocate the turbulence in my breath, but I didn't have the strength. I couldn't silence the sounds. I lied naked in the fetal position, feeling my cabin cave in like a collapsing womb. I roared into my pillow once more, calling out for God to save me from this panic attack, but god had no place in the hell I had put myself in. Once my breathing slowed down, I rolled over to the ladder and stumbled onto the floor. My chest bent over my knees as I grabbed the back of my head, curling tightly into a ball, as it was the only way I knew how to make myself small.

Placing my hands on the cold carpet, it took all my might to push myself to kneel. One foot at a time, I stood to grab hold of my bunk's railing, feeling the ship rock despite being docked on calm waters. I shuffled back into the bathroom, noticing just a little food left in the toilet. It took one more flush for my excretion to vanish, followed by a wipe and a rinse to clean up the residue.

I stepped into the shower to cleanse me of the filth that I was and the mess that I had made. My panic attack dwindled down, but the aftershock had only just begun. Dripping out of the shower, I pulled my towel from its ring to rub out the disgust that sunk deep below my skin. As hard as it was to look at myself in the mirror, I knew I needed to pull myself together before I would die across international waters.

It took me another ten minutes to collect my breath and call Molly. I requested a meeting with her as soon as possible and she agreed to meet in the gallery just an hour before we opened that afternoon.

"Molly, I'm not well." I sat facing her in our lowly-lit gallery, sitting on opposite sides of the desk. Molly's big eyes widened even more, like she was waiting for a plot to implode in a drama series.

"I'm depressed. Really depressed. I'm not myself here, and I don't feel like I'm able to work at the caliber I could be if I wasn't so stressed. I don't feel like I'm fitting in, and HR continues to pair me with a new roommate each week, which is taking a toll on my sense of stability." A wave of relief came over me as I pleaded to leave.

"I know, Jenny. We can all tell something isn't right." Molly switched her commanding tone to a promising one, as she was about to sign off on my resignation.

"I am so sorry, but I don't think I can finish up this last month of my contract." I admitted.

"It's ok, Jenny. We suspected something was going on. But no need to explain, Lewis and I will talk to corporate tonight and get you home when we reach Florida on Friday." Molly smiled, and for the first time in five months, offered a hug. Though it felt forced, human touch was what my body craved, and all I needed to recuperate for my final days on board.

I spent the next few nights alone, numbing out on food and booze, too exhausted to care about my health. I had rapidly put on 20 pounds over the past month, hardly squeezing into elastic size 6 pants, figuring, 'why stop now' when I still had buffets at my disposal. While the promise of returning home should have lifted a weight off my shoulders, I resented myself for giving up on my job instead. Despite my stigma towards quitting, I had to leave. I knew if I did not, I could die at sea.

On my last night on the Bella Fiesta, Lewis and Molly asked the team to watch movies in their larger cabin, drink Johnnie Walker Black Label and say goodbye to the gallery director. Obligated, I complied to socialize over my ardent desire to spend my last hours by the late-night pizza parlor. I pretended to laugh at their jokes when Lewis pointed out, "Jenny, I reckon you're not that excited to go home, are you sure you don't want to stay?" he teased.

My expression could not hide the dread in my face. I was too tired for excitement and too checked out to pretend to care.

"Oh, I suppose it's bittersweet." I said sheepishly. This forced camaraderie was ending. I wondered what my career on ships would have looked like if I had expressed my concerns to HR and requested a transfer to another team. Because on the Queen Pearl, I adored my colleagues like family. Here, I was the black sheep.

"I just miss home." I said as a safe response to an offhand question.

...

When my brother picked me up from the airport, he sat stoned in the driver's seat as he watched me load my luggage into the trunk, though his staggered stare wasn't from the weed.

Confused, he turned to me before we drove back home.

"I didn't recognize you, Jenny."

I know he wanted to show support, but he didn't know how. My weight gain was rapid and pulled me down into a new degree of depression. I had lost the spark in my eyes; I had lost the spirit in my step. I hollowed myself during that year on ships to stay afloat; chasing status more than I did the sale. I had told friends, family, and guests on the ship about how much I *"loved my job,"* because I didn't want to seem unappreciative while sailing across the Caribbean. These fallacies dug me into a deeper hole of deception, leaving me to binge to fill the void. I may have retired from an opportunity to work upon the seven seas, but I wasn't about to give up travel just yet.

The Trip of a Lifetime

When living in Florence, my girlfriends and I would clink our glasses and salute to being "fat, broke, and happy." When I returned to Kansas after resigning from cruise ships, I was just fat. Fat in my eyes, at least, having gained fifty pounds in eighteen months. Where my self-worth and tolerance for the mirror were at an all-time low, my checking account was the largest it had ever been. Nearing five figures to my name, I opted out from a savings account and "invested in myself." If I wanted a life of freedom and exploration, I'd need a proper brand like the travel bloggers I'd idealized over the years. The Blogger site I started while studying abroad wouldn't do, I'd need a polished website with my own dotcom. I'd want a bigger reach than my number one fan who, of course, was my grandma. Grandma believed in my abilities to make it as a travel writer. So, I went for it.

Choosing the first link that popped up on a Google search, I hired two male designers in Kansas City to help me develop my site, "Live Prolific." With no sponsors or endorsements, investors, or sugar daddies to fund this venture of documenting my travels, my best course of action would have been to build a site on my own for less than $100. But I was impatient, immature, and painfully naive, and instead dropped a grand in the hands of the two dudes in KC who (in hindsight) totally took advantage of me. After our brief consultation, I hired them to create a logo which I loathed and looked like a construction site's emblem, but I was too ashamed to pull back after paying an invoice upfront. Alas, after two weeks of correspondence, liveprolific.com was up and running and I now possessed 1,000 business cards and 100 magnets that I would give out to less than ten people who already had my phone number.

One lucky recipient of a Live Prolific magnet was my grandma. She and a few other aunts were the only family I had that celebrated my writing and saw it as a possible career, validating my dreams of being compensated for my excursions. But other prominent members of the Martin household, along with peers and acquaintances from the Midwest did not view writing as a viable vocation.

"Jenny Martin! What are you up to these days?" An old pal would ask whilst having a run in at a bar.

"I'm a freelancer." I'd say to my fellow comrade.

"Freelancing what?" the chap would speculate.

"Writing." I'd say in liquid confidence.

"So… what do you do for money?" the wee lad would probe.

"I work!" I'd exclaim without explanation and scatter off.

Several people in my circles raised suspicion as to how I was able to travel so extensively. No, I didn't have a wealthy husband and no, I didn't have a trust fund. Though I imagined this was the case for how some travel bloggers got their start after crossing stunning accounts of bleached blondes on Instagram. I was determined to make it as a blogger and label my posts as "sponsored." But to be a travel blogger, one must travel. So, I called up my gal pals from Florence and arranged another trip to Europe to be with the dream team from 2013.

Cher, my bubbly, long-haired, blonde friend from California was now working for EuroTour and insisted I crash in her Italian apartment. Brooklyn, who had interned with EuroTour, also received an extension of this invitation, as she too was between jobs and longing for another skip across the pond.

With money to blow and a professional website to archive it all, I flew to Florence to meet Cher and Brooklyn in September of 2015 for a week of reminiscing, wine, and a crap top of cheese. I wouldn't be squandering like the last time, and I certainly wouldn't take any abuse by an Italian this time - or so I told myself.

It dawned on me that in the three times I had visited Florence, Brooklyn always seemed to arrive by my side, establishing a sense of security in a fabulously foreign city. With no worries of a job back home, we weaved around the majestic Duomo, basking in its glory. We sat outside on a cafe patio overlooking the infamous, red-tiled dome with our iPads and books, unbothered by street merchants peddling us silk scarves as we sipped espresso, reading and writing on the cobblestone streets. Brooklyn dove her head into fiction, whereas I typed out a fantasy version of how I was experiencing Italy on my blog. Always writing about where to go, reluctant to share how I was truly feeling; *lost*.

On our second day, Brooklyn insisted we find a CrossFit class so she could stay consistent with the training she followed back home. To me, Brooklyn had always looked fit and confident in her skin. Though it was apparent by her newly cinched waist that she had drank the barbell Kool-Aid. Because of the results I saw in Brooklyn, I agreed to bus 30 minutes outside of Florence for a workout. And thankfully I agreed, as I had a blast beating out burpees and batting eyes at our curly haired coach. Overall, I got a hit of endorphins which prompted me to catch more feel-good vibes all night long.

Cher, Brooklyn, and I dolled up after the gym, swapping wardrobes and reminiscing on the good 'ol study abroad days. Our trio went out before a weekend split, where Brooklyn and I would scurry off to Budapest while Cher worked a EuroTour trip. Returning to our hub at Kikuya, we drank until my eyes rolled back into my head, which oddly took only one Dragoon. I soon slipped out of Kikuya with a cute Italian man to continue a conversation as he lit a cigarette. But sometime after leaving my friends, I found myself pinned against a wall between three or four men. Their hands grabbed up and between my legs. They took turns pecking at my neck as I looked up to the streetlights, flaccid and helpless. The only face I could shape was the one I met at Kikuya, whom I intended to join just for a cigarette. But shortly after leaving the bar, every *body* - including mine - became a blur, and the night became one big regret.

I was now in a fetal position, dressed and distressed against a random doorstep. Panicking and patting for my purse. My cash was intact, but my phone was as dead as the night. I was aware enough to direct myself back to Cher's apartment, though when I rang the bell, no one was awake to answer.

I pounded for minutes before a familiar voice called from afar.

"Jenny!" Brooklyn cried.

Thank God. Brooklyn sent a message to Cher before *her* phone died. We gave up knocking and curled up on the curb, burrowing our heads on top of one another. We were cold, drunk, laughing and crying on the streets, waiting for rescue. And just as I drifted off into a slumber, my head swung back as Cher cracked open the door.

Sunshine creeped through the wooden shades of Cher's apartment, rudely awakening two hungover Americans in a vacant Italian apartment. I noticed Cher's empty bed and checked the clock:

9:38 AM

Fack!

Brooklyn and I had thirty minutes to catch our train to Rome before our budget flight to Budapest. Frantic, I started throwing toiletries and underwear from my suitcase into a duffel bag, ripping off my dress from our night out to change into something suitable for the plane.

"Brooklyn!" I shrieked. She was still rolling in bed.

"Jenny, doll. Don't worry. We still have plenty of time to catch the train."

"No, Brooklyn, come here... *look.*"

Our eyes drew towards my crotch, now dabbed in a halo of bruises circling my inner thighs and lower abdomen.

"Jenny..." Brooklyn's tone lowered with concern. "Were you...?"

Vague shadows of towering men clouded my thinking. My head was pounding, and I thought and thought and thought. But I couldn't answer Brooklyn, so I asked myself... *was I?*

"No, I wasn't." I said to placate the possibility that I could have been.

"But Brooklyn, I only drank half a pint of Dragoon. And that was after a big dinner. There's no reason I should have gotten so drunk."

"Same, Jen. After just one drink, I don't remember *anything.* I just remember losing you then losing Cher. Then forgetting my way home - which has *never* happened to me in Florence. I don't think we got drunk last night. I think we were drugged." Brooklyn said soberly.

My head swelled. I drowned in guilt. Did we just get roofied? Did I just get r— sexually assaulted? This must have meant that I was the one to blame. I put myself into this dangerous position with my promiscuity, so eager to drink and so easily taken advantage of. I shook it off, telling myself it wasn't a big deal because I wasn't raped, just felt up, grabbed, and kissed while unconscious. Besides, who would I report to? And who would I report? I had no name, no face, no number... only a ring of bruises around my privates. So, I kept it private. I would have to bear the shame and resurface the pain for a different day. Because that morning, Brooklyn and I had a train to catch.

I hoped to leave my remorse in Florence, that the faint memories of the evening would pass over me like the tunnels we coursed through on the high-speed Trenitalia. But as Brooklyn caught up on sleep in the seat next to me, unanswered questions ran rapidly in my head.

When did I start fading out? When did I meet the Italian man? Why did I agree to leave with him and his posse of strange men? At which moment did the flirting turn forceful? Was I submissive? Was I a slut? Does drunken silence count as consent? Will this keep happening?

I thought I had used my sexuality for power. Power over attention, power through attraction. I had drawn this Italian man in with a single stare, letting him know he'd met his match. But little did I know, I was the one who had caught the bait. The edges of my memory reveal his smile from across the bar, then his smile much closer to my face. Somewhere between 'ciao' and curling up on the curb with Brooklyn, my sexual power was stripped away, manipulated, and turned against me.

With a couple of hours to spare in Rome, Brooklyn and I kept close to the train station, finding a quaint, quiet place for lunch. We plopped our luggage and our tired bones into the wooden seats, ordering pizza and drinking Peroni's over white tablecloths. Brooklyn and I ate slowly, speaking even slower. Songs of the streets filled our lack of dialogue. We did not force conversation. We could just be silent. We could just be.

This peace was interrupted by two middle-aged American couples, laughing and drunk before their wine arrived. One woman peeked over her shoulder and down at our bags to ask, "first time in Italy?" Brooklyn and I smiled at each other like honeymooners in bliss. Or our eyes were still sunken from sleep deprivation.

"No, not our first time. But we did meet in Italy. Is this your first time?" I asked, staring at their freshly printed "ROMA" tee-shirts.

"O yes! We are celebrating our 25th wedding anniversary and invited our friends along for the ride. This is all our first time in Europe. It's been the trip of a lifetime. And you! You ladies are so young and have already been to Italy! You're so lucky."

Smiling in reciprocation, I immediately regretted my eyeroll at the start of the conversation, as the "trip of a lifetime" line was one of which I found so limiting. But who was I to judge? I was just some young, single white girl who prioritized travel over a savings account, whereas people my age were starting to get married and house hunt. That was *their* dream. Just because my life made for a pretty online page, did not make my aspirations any better or noble than settling down.

Luckily for me, Brooklyn was in a similar nomadic stage that September when we landed in Budapest. While strolling across riverside skylines overlooking rolling hills and Gothic architecture, we took walking tours and pub crawls and even stumbled upon a wine festival on top of a castle. However, our main objective for this Hungarian trip was attending the 'sparty' at the Széchenyi Spas. This attraction is the largest medicinal bath in Europe, with twenty-one pools, ten hot baths, saunas, and wellness services. Though on the weekends when the sun goes down, the strobe lights come out along with hundreds of horny men wading through warm waters.

I had lofty expectations for the Sparty, as former friends had described their experience as *euphoric*. But as Saturday progressed, my sweet Brooklyn was still hungover from the previous night's pub crawl. While primping for the Sparty, I was worried whether Brooklyn would hold her liquor better than she held down breakfast. However, I was mostly concerned about how I looked in my swimsuit. Back home, everyone knew me as "the skinny friend." So, when the "skinny friend" gained weight, I carried more burdens on my shoulders than I did a pudge around my waist. But here in Budapest, where I *only* knew Brooklyn, it dawned on me that I did not have to be "the skinny girl who gained weight," I could be *whoever I wanted to be*. And what a relief. Yet that cognitive relief switched to grief when I looked at myself in the mirror. Lifting my bottoms, scooping up my tits, sucking in my belly - I tried all the tricks. I would then turn to the side, horrified, grab a swig of my beer, and say, "fuck it."

At least I gained boobs. I sighed to myself. After leaving the Bella Fiesta, I spent two months vigorously exercising and undereating, shedding about fifteen pounds from my highest weight, still forty away from my lowest. While I had mastered the art of layering loose clothing between those pounds, there was nothing I could hide in a two-piece swimsuit.

"Are you ready, Brooklyn?" I asked as I grabbed my purse and jacket, hoping she would hurry up. My big boobs and my eager ass could not wait to get drunk again, swim in the spas, and see what the hype of the magic baths were all about. After a 20-minute cab ride through the sparkling metropolis, we arrived at the palace-like entrance of the Széchenyi spas. Depositing our belongings in the locker room, we stepped out into the cool September night, watching steam reflect off the blue and red disco lights surrounding the vicinity. The various pools reached far past our scope of vision, but the bar was near in sight. Sober and insecure about the width of my waist, I confidently stepped up to the bartender and assured myself that liquor would melt away any of my body woes. When I turned to give Brooklyn her vodka tonic, she was nowhere in sight.

How could I have lost her already? I'm too sober to stand alone in a swimsuit!

Behind a tall, chiseled silhouette, I spotted my friend talking to someone with immaculate butt dimples. Walking up with our drinks, I was invisible to the intense eye-contact between Brooklyn and this strange man, a link that could only be severed by a cock block.

"Here you go." I jutted her cocktail out, expecting Brooklyn to introduce me to this man and most importantly, his friends.

It took a sentence or two for Brooklyn and Johnny Bravo to acknowledge the friend who had so graciously waited in line for a whole two minutes to deliver drinks. I stood there smiling, shifting my weight from hip to hip, miming, "look at me!" while waiting for their attention.

"Jenny, this is Stephan."

Stephan turned towards me to extend a sculpted arm, draped in tattoos.

"Pleasure," Stephan said in a soft, English accent.

An Englishman?! Damn. Brooklyn's weak spot.

"Jenny! Stephan is on holiday from Bath and owns a CrossFit gym. How funny is that?"

An Englishman who owns a CrossFit. That's fucking hilarious.

"Who would have guessed?" I smiled forcefully while clasping my drink, which was now suddenly empty.

I left Brooklyn and Stephan to flirt as I continued drinking and drifting between other traveling females. I followed a tall, red-headed woman with a delightful English accent into the spas, where she introduced me to a half dozen men sporting booty-clenching briefs, bow ties and sailor hats. One sailor caught my eye while wading waist-deep in the pool. His name was Freddy.

"How's business?" I asked Freddy.

"Excuse me?" He responded in yet again, another English accent.

"Stripping!" I tapped the tip of his hat.

"Back in the States, strippers make a killing." I smiled.

Freddy smiled, but not too wide.

"Ya, it's just a side gig for now, to get me through veterinary school."

"Veterinary school? You have a soft spot for animals?" I pursed my lips together.

"Kittens" He purred.

"Strippers and kittens" I purred back.

"Strippers and kittens." His smile widened as he leaned into me.

"I gather you're not all strippers, so what's with the matching outfits? I said as I pulled away from the kiss.

"My mate is getting married. We're here for his stag party."

"Like a bachelor party?" I asked.

"Like a bachelor party," he said.

"Damn. I was really hoping you were a stripper. And let me guess" I said, "You're not studying to be a vet."

"That part is true. Because I do love…" Freddy leaned in to press his lips up to mine.

"Kittens."

If Freddy wasn't a vet, then he could have been an Abercrombie model, chiseled from all angles. Handsome, with a shyness about him. He acted nervous and a bit aloof between electric charges of face grabbing. I couldn't help but feel something was off, but instead of listening to my insecurities, I let them drift into the gutter. Thoughts of "you're too fat for him" were banished each time Freddy took my hand to dance. My drunken confidence told this conniving voice that if my physique were a cockblock, then Freddy would have never kissed me in the first place. I kept tricking myself - because it was so damn hard to believe - that someone would choose me among the hundreds of other girls who were far, far skinnier.

Could this mean that I was still desirable with the extra weight I had gained since college? Or was my personality bigger than my body… or was I just a pretty face? Pondering this, Freddy left my side to converse with his friends. I sighed. *Must be the big boobs.*

With hundreds of nearly naked bodies still swimming through the steamy venue, the party was ending. Drunk and horny, I became impatient in guessing where it would lead. Then, a few of Freddy's mates came up to me when Freddy was away, probing about our apparent connection.

"What do you think of Freddy?" They asked.

"Well, he checks my only boxes, being British and a good swimmer." The friends laughed, catching Freddy's attention from across the pool.

"You seem pretty cool." One of the friends egged me on as I tried to figure out where this conversation was going.

"Freddy's a great guy. But he's had some girl issues in the past, you know? It would be nice to see him with someone chill like you."

I laughed. Freddy was hot. Abercrombie hot. But what were his friends playing at? Long distance? *Mmm… no thank you.* But a 12-hour love affair, that I could sustain.

The DJ announced the last call to a pool packed with young lovers. Freddy returned to kiss me, then let his gaze drift away. I shot him a look that read, *"you're not telling me something."* Then point blank, I asked, "what?"

Freddy took in a long inhale and sighed it out.

"Jenny, I am in a relationship, an ending one. She's been my girlfriend for four years…but…"

My eyes widened as I anticipated what was coming next.

"But I really want to fuck you."

I felt a release of anxiety flow out from his body as he admitted this, still holding on tightly to my waist.

"Well," I waited for his eyes to focus onto mine. "What are you waiting for?"

…

Retrieving my dress and purse from the locker, I knew there was no point in finding Brooklyn as we agreed non-verbally at the start of the Sparty that she would be going home with Stephan. I found Freddy waiting for me in the queue of cabs, ready to rock his world, for one night only.

Morning came, expiring our short shelf life of time together. I dressed quickly and carefully, trying to gain a sense of innocence after a primitive act. Freddy held my hand as he walked me to the hotel entrance. He kept his gaze forward, afraid to show the guilt in his eyes. When we reached the front doors, he looked down to give me our final kiss.

"Goodbye, Jenny." He leaned down onto me.

"Take care." I said, leaving to hail a cab, and never looked back.

…

On my ride back to grab Brooklyn from our hostel, I pulled my chlorinated, sweat-soaked sex hair into a bun while watching the eclectic architecture of Budapest pass by. Entering our room, four feet hung off the top bunk of the beds.

"Heeeey beebee" I cooed.

"It's 9am. We only have a few hours until our flight. Let's pack up and grab breakfast."

Brooklyn peeled her head off Stephan's bare chest, smiling childishly as she opened her eyes.

"Hi... Hey... Ya ok..."

Nothing registered.

"Brookie babe, I'm going to start packing for you. What do you want to wear on the plane?"

I threw our belongings together and left out a spare outfit for Brooklyn, if she ever decided to get dressed.

"I'm heading downstairs to check us out, let's leave in the next ten." I warned her, hoping she would follow my lead.

I stood by the hostel corridor anxiously, wondering if my tapping foot would echo back up the stairs and into the room where I left Brooklyn and Stephan.

Why did I leave them alone again? Poor choice on my part. At least there are other guests sleeping in the room. She wouldn't have the indecency to start at it aga....

"We're ready!" Brooklyn said minutes later. She tiptoed down the stairs with a purse in one hand and Stephan's grip in the other. Her face was so smitten, and he was so sure of himself. While I was happy for Brooklyn, I wasn't all too excited about this dude clinging onto my friend.

"Cool... so there's a market on the way to the airport. I figured we could walk around a little and get something to eat." And when I said *"we"* I meant me and Brooklyn.

A cab slowed down and drove up to the curb, popping its trunk for us to load in our luggage. I sat behind the driver as I waited for Stephan to release my friend, then shook my head in disbelief when the two joined me in the back seat.

God damn! He's a lingerer.

Stephan paid the driver. Which was aggravating because it gave me one less reason to loathe him.

We ordered breakfast from an outdoor patio, and I begrudgingly hid my resentment around the newest addition of our girl's weekend. To my disappointment, Stephan was charming, kind, and kinda cool. This mitigated my pettiness, but I still craved one-on-one time with Brooklyn to unload the events of last night. Afterall, I wasn't going to tell some *strange man* that I had slept with a *taken man*! I'm no homewrecker, Stephan. You don't know me.

After savory crepes and fresh squeezed orange juice, our little group grazed an open market of crafts and artwork, picking up last minute gifts for ourselves and our friends back home. Finally, I told Brooklyn I would wait for her at the end of the street so she and Stephan could say their goodbyes as I hailed a cab.

Alone, I contemplated the possibility of long-distance relationships within this short life span and came to the consensus: "what's the point?" Brooklyn then skidded up next to me with a wide smile, eager to share secrets and sex stories.

"I'm going to see him!" She exclaimed.

"See who?" I asked facetiously.

"To see Stephan!" She kept smiling, bug-eyed.

"But you just saw Stephan. If you look close enough, you can still see him on the street corner." I pointed behind us jokingly, but I couldn't seem to shake the love spell off Brooklyn's face.

"I'm changing my flights home as soon as we're connected to Wi-Fi." She said.

Damn.

"At least one of us got oral last night." I sighed as Brooklyn blushed.

"Jenny!"

When Brookyln and I said our goodbyes, I headed to Kansas while she changed her flights. Landing in Bath, England, Brooklyn soon found out that Stephan's missing roommate was in fact his ex-wife, who flipped when she came home to see Brooklyn's suitcase in the living room. Stephan tried covering up by saying 'they were over,' and that 'she's hardly home.' But Brooklyn didn't buy into his bullshit and found acquaintances to crash with in London as all that sweet love making turned sour *real* quick.

...

The minute I returned home to Kansas, I devised my next move. While my *Live Prolific* page was increasing in posts, the site's engagement still derived from friends and family. Less than 100 page views wouldn't commission a sponsored article, but that wasn't driving me to write. I genuinely enjoyed engineering words onto a page as a product of my experience. Though when I returned home from Budapest, I couldn't depend on my writing career to take off and sustain me. If I wanted to keep a free room at my parents, I needed a job that was, as they like to say, *"realistic."*

"Ok, I've made a decision. I know what I'm going to do." I announced at dinner only days after arriving back from Budapest. My parents kept their eyes locked on their plates, dreading the news of my next international antic.

"I'm going to teach English in Korea." I shined my teeth, hoping my enthusiasm would rub off on the rest of the table. Not to my surprise though still to my disappointment, my parent's reactions were less than thrilled.

"Which Korea?" My dad asked in horror.

"Which one do you think?" I blew back.

"But Jenny, what about your eating? Do you really think it's a good idea to go so far away when you're still having problems with food?" My dad's frustrated face started to redden. "You can't just run away from your disease." He said.

"I know, and I'm not. I haven't thrown up since the ships. The sales job was too stressful for me, it was… fueling my bulimia. Also, the buffets on the ships were so unhealthy. Besides, I don't like Korean food, so I won't have anything to binge on." I pleaded.

"Have you ever tried Korean food?" My mom asked.

"No, have *you* ever tried Korean food?" I shot back.

"This isn't about me. This is about your health." Mom said.

"Koreans are like, so skinny and healthy!" I exclaimed.

My parents nodded their heads in agreement to that.

"But why Korea, Jenny?" My mom asked, flabbergasted.

"Well, I've spent the past 48-hours researching teaching opportunities, and Korea offers the most lucrative salary without needing an education degree. Plus, it's a progressive, safe, collective culture. I want a break from the individualistic mindsets of America and other Western countries. I want to live in Asia. I want to be surrounded in symbols I can't read. I want a challenge."

My parents rolled their eyes as I could hardly see through the glaze in mine.

"Oh, you'll get your challenge." Dad said.

With a couple months to spare before my Asian adventure and very little savings left from the cruise ships, I moved to Florida with my retired dad over the winter. He is a snowbird in the Sunshine State for the colder half of the year, then migrates back to Kansas for the summer. My mom joined us sporadically, flying between states, working part-time as a nurse in the winters.

185

To save up, I juggled shifts at a J. Crew with waitressing at a large sports bar. Yet I still made time to tan by the pool, visit the beach and work out. And my latest exercise of choice? *CrossFit.* I decided to drink the juice and join a "box" that was a short bike ride from my parent's condo. In that hour each day, I felt powerful, competitive, and strong in my skin. Though all too often, my dedication to obtain a certain shape would rev up a hunger within, and I'd end up eating more than I burned in my WOD. (Work out of the day.)

My dad, though reluctant to say much, showed his support by dropping me off at work as I was dependent on him for a car. During one ride back from my dinner shift, my dad addressed a viable concern.

"Do you have any apprehensions about moving, Jenny?" he asked unexpectedly. He was never one to bring up Asia.

"Any apprehensions?" I asked, wondering where this was coming from. I had already traveled so much - what did either of us have to worry about?

"About your eating." He said sternly.

I diverted my eyes away from his, to think honestly about my eating from the past few months. Physically, I looked strong. But as I exercised, I ate. I wrestled with paleo diets while sneaking out for donuts and ice cream. I frequently asked my dad to drop me off at Starbucks before shifts, stocking up on cake pops and croissants without his knowing. When I wasn't working, I would bike to a bakery, binge on an assortment of Danishes and throw it all up behind a bush on the ride home. I tried limiting binging and purging to once a week, with exceptions. Every day, I obsessed over food and exercising, always canceling out the two. So much of the money I was making was spent on food, and each gluttonous receipt filed through my mind as I exhaled and responded to my father.

"I mean… I don't see myself having a problem with food in Korea. I'll be so consumed with the culture change and the responsibilities of my new job, that I won't really be phased by food. Plus, having a routine as a teacher will help with my eating and workout schedule."

While I wanted to believe my words, I realized how naive I sounded: *I plan to escape my problems, to a country where my eating disorder can't catch me.*

My dad studied the traffic light ahead. I knew his bland expression meant that a web of worry was spinning through his head. We sat silently for a few minutes, until we reached our driveway.

"I want you to consider a meeting." He said.

By meeting, he meant a 12-step meeting. Like the Alcoholics Anonymous meetings which saved his life over thirty years ago. My dad and I rarely talked about addiction, and even more rarely brought up his. But to show his concern about our shared genetic makeup was to show his guarded love for me. My eyes watered up as I nodded in agreement. We both knew that the greatest lie an addict can make is not in a manipulative plot to deceive another, but in the lie they tell themselves that they can fight their inner demons on their own.

Stepping through the stale church doors turned a warm, sunny morning into a day which would leave me cold for weeks. Expecting enlightenment, I instead watched the room dim into black and white. Members filed in and greeted each other kindly, some more happy to be there than others. I was the youngest one in the room by a few decades and the thinnest person by a few hundred pounds. I cringed during the recitation of the opening prayer.

Is this where my future lies? I wondered.

A closet of elastic pants and a walking cane?

I listened fearfully as the members shared stories and hope for their disease. Looking around in disbelief, I fast forwarded my own life into a pair of their shoes and imagined eating relentlessly every step of the way.

O shit, it's my turn.

"I'm Jenny, and I'm a compulsive overeater."

I hadn't really paid attention to the other speakers, as each anecdote reminded me too much of myself. I had averted my attention back inside, thinking: *Maybe I'm not alone in this compulsion to eat, but I sure as hell don't want to end up like them.* I couldn't say this out loud, of course. But I did convey something I thought the room would appreciate, which, for years, had been stored safely in my mind.

"I came to this meeting as a suggestion from my dad, who is a recovering alcoholic. His sobriety has helped him for over thirty years, so I figured if this works for him, it might work for me. But the thing with drinking is that it leads to inebriation, it inhibits you from driving, working, or whatever. With eating, no one really knows when you're in a binge except for you. Sure, a food coma can leave you foggy and lethargic. Though sometimes I wish I had a drinking problem instead; it would feel less shameful than admitting that I binge on food as my fix."

I paused as I locked eyes with members of the group, many of whom were nodding in agreement.

"When I was anorexic, I used to dream of the day I'd get pregnant and old, as I told myself that those would be the only times in my life I'd allow myself to overeat."

Another pause. Not for dramatic effect, but because what I was saying had been locked inside for so long, it took me another breath to let it out.

"If I could eat whatever I wanted without the consequence of gaining weight, I would binge every day. I would feast for breakfast, lunch, and dinner, without a vegetable in sight. This is what I dream about all day and night and yet, and I'd kill for the cravings to go away. I'll do anything to not give in. But I always do. And that's why I'm here... Thank you."

One last pause. My eyes burned through the welcome packet that laid on the table in front of me. The room responded with a unanimous "thank you" and "we're glad you're here." But I couldn't hear them. I spaced out for the rest of that meeting while anticipating my visit to the closest bakery that I could catch on my drive home with the car I borrowed from my dad.

Expressing my gluttonous desires to a room of people who shared my same twisted cravings was a bit relieving, but this confession didn't fix anything; it only unleashed the truth of who I was. Admitting myself as "Jenny, compulsive overeater," permitted me to not only see myself as an addict, but to live as one. This initial meeting was a turning point in my disease down a tumultuous road of recovery.

...

Fun fact: Drinking is an integrated aspect of Korean culture. Drugs are not. The repercussions and societal shame one may endure if caught with drugs in Korea are so vast, that I decided to ingest whatever substances I could before a year of drug-free living. Now, a drug test was scheduled during my first few weeks in Korea for a health screening, but the beauty of a pee test is that most substances are cleared from your system in a matter of days apart from my favorite recreational fix, marijuana.

I quit the ganga exactly one month before my flight to Seoul, giving my body ample time to sweat out cannabinoids under the Floridian sun. But when one of my server friends from the restaurant asked if I was interested in tripping mushrooms with her during my last weekend in Florida, I said "groovy."

My server friend Becca was a college student living with her roommate Ashley in Estero, where we would *do the drugs*. The three of us blended the fungi into orange juice and sucked down the shrooms while setting our intentions for the trip. Becca asked for guidance in her career, and Ashley sought healing from a long streak of anxiety and depression. I grabbed my fortified juice with both hands, seeking peace and promise as I entered a new chapter in my life. The bits of mushrooms trickled down my throat. It would take another hour for still life to start moving, but we didn't waste any time.

Ashley played The Beatles on surround speakers and laid out yoga mats for the three of us in the living room. She led us through a flow as the psychedelics began to seep through our system, until we freestyled to our own beat during the come up.

We were together and alone at once, feeling the medicine move through our bodies, creating new pathways in our minds. My hosts laid out art supplies, assembling acrylics on paper plates to explore colors on a blank canvas. There was no need for brushes, as fingertips served as the best tool for my masterpiece.

After completing a landscape of waves and polka-dots, I expanded the art onto my body. Every touch of my finger graced my limbs with care, and I watched in awe as a dot of blue paint cooled my skin and released a river of hues as it swam before my eyes. I wasn't making art. I was art.

Once our designs dried, the three of us took a ladder to their shallow rooftop. Not the smartest idea, but it seemed fitting at the time. Laying on a blanket, the clouds passed us like angels floating above our heads. Then, Becca said something that I'll never forget:

"God did this."

We laid paralyzed with insight before breaking into laughing tears. I had been questioning my belief in God for some time now, though this euphoric rush of boundless wonder seemed possible because of some kind of grand creator.

"Yes, Becca. *God* did this." I gasped.

There were no lows during this high. There were only moments of silent, inner solitude woven between childish cheers. When the mushrooms began to wear off, we started "The Secret Life of Walter Mitty," a Ben Stiller film based on a short story by James Thurber. The fantastic tale follows a man living in fear that he will never be good enough to achieve the relationships or experiences he desires, and thus sleepwalks at work while daydreaming his life away. But when Mitty's job at *Life* magazine is jeopardized, he embarks on the adventure of a lifetime.

As the movie ended, so did our trip. When Becca turned to me near the end of the film to ask, "are you ready?" she was, of course, referring to my new life in Korea. This was a question I was afraid the mushrooms would tantalize me with during the high, as I was stepping into a world unknown. I ultimately ate the shrooms in confidence, ready to face a potential "bad trip" if that's what the mushrooms wanted me to endure. But all I felt was wonder and ecstasy. I looked to Becca in confidence and replied:

"Yea. I'm ready."

When the drugs wore off, I felt slightly less ready though cocky for sure. I stepped on my transpacific flight the next week with even less conviction, but there was no turning back. Just like eating magic mushrooms or dropping a tab of acid, you never really know what to expect on your trip. I was taking the same gamble with my life, though instead of the drugs wearing off in 12 hours, I subjected myself to this episode for the next 365 days of my life.

I craved change through an external source as the inside job seemed a lot harder than teaching English in Asia. Besides, another move would prove to myself and others that I was independent and could make it on my own. So what if I had a little eating disorder? Surely it couldn't follow me to Korea. My decision to move to a new continent in a country that spoke a different language working in a career that I had zero experience in among a metropolitan where I knew no one would be good for me... *right*?

The Seoul Solution

There is something in the ventilation system on airplanes that puts me right to sleep. Or perhaps it is the acceleration from lift off - the gravitational pull that jerks me back into my seat, rocking me so deep. Whatever it may be, my hidden talent of sleeping soundly on planes was suppressed during that 12-hour flight to South Korea. I hadn't slept more than four hours a night leading up to the move, as each minute I inched closer to my life in Korea, time disclosed that this decision was final. There was no going back.

I landed in Seoul's Incheon International Airport around 36am, which is not a time, but rather a space into which I entered after traveling across time zones. I could comprehend that it was dark, I was tired, and until I connected to a Wi-Fi spot, I had no way of communicating with my new boss who planned to pick me up upon landing.

Luckily for me, Koreans are collectively warm people, so the first person I asked was open to lending me a phone to contact my school principal, Sunny. I found Sunny through a Canadian recruiting service online after a weekend of intense research and internal debates over what I was doing with my life. The Canadians then paired me with a Korean recruiter as a translator, who in turn connected me with Sunny. After a full five-minute conversation of broken English and basic questions about my experience with children, the school offered me the position. For the first time in my evolving career, I scored the job without a plug. And that felt like a big accomplishment. Never mind the ease and immediacy of this hire. I was much too psyched from the green light that I ignored any red flags.

My plan was foolproof. Or dare I say, *golden*. The hagwon, or private kindergarten center, would pay for my rent, my flight to Korea, and a comfortable salary of two million won, which comes to roughly $1,750 USD per month. I would not be raining in won, but I would get by. Besides, I had always "gotten by," so how would this be any different?

Pacing around the arrivals lane in my purple puffer, I carried life by the handles. Two suitcases and a backpack, to be exact. I waited. I wondered. I started to worry. Was I in the right lane? Would my new boss spot the only blonde girl in the Incheon Airport? After an hour of bobbing around like an NPC, I noticed a yellow school van turn onto the pick-up lane.

"Welcome Jen-eee!" Sunny jumped out of the van, smiling wide as her jet-black bob swung side to side. A white woman stepped out behind her.

"Hello, Welcome to Korea." said the current English teacher, Tess, in a somber tone. Tess looked as tired as I did, despite my jetlag.

After this short exchange, we drove an hour through the night between the electric metropolitan. Seoul is home to over ten million, compressing one fifth of the nation's population into a country the size of Iowa. Yet, I refrained from speaking to the first two people I met in Korea, too wiped with jet lag to start small talk. Sunny and Tessa didn't seem to mind, as we all gazed at the jungle of skyscrapers on our ride into town. Bridge after bridge, we flew above the dark waters of Seoul's major streams. These black breaks in the road looked like a mirage from my window, projecting a warped reflection from the neon lights of the city.

We stopped in Yongin, a smaller city of 1 million just south of Seoul. But unlike the four, five, and six bedroom homes that reside in suburban neighborhoods back in the Midwest, this suburb felt no different than the city center we just passed. Less skyscrapers, but still a condensed, high-rise collection of modern buildings. Sunny helped me unload my luggage to my shoebox apartment on the third floor, gave me a hug and in her best English said, "See you Wednesday!"

Tess stayed behind to give me a tour around the 200-square-foot apartment she was handing off. As Tess downsized and stayed at a friend's during this transitional week, she graciously left me a blow dryer, a drying rack, and a kitchen stocked with a pot and a pan for the stove top. There was no microwave or oven. There was, however, a utility closet, a table, a single chair, and a twin bed with no box spring. Still, bigger than a ship's cabin, and a room I could call my own. *Home sweet home.*

Luckily, I had arrived on the Monday night before election day, which is a national holiday in Korea and a day off for the hagwon. Tess suggested I use the free time to prepare for Wednesday's class and buy groceries. After all, I was diving headfirst into a new field without any formal training. There would be no orientation, no study guide. Just me, the internet, and three short days of shadowing.

Tess shut the door behind her, solidifying my solitude in this foreign country. The rush of fascination and awe I had anticipated for months never manifested. I looked at my measly mattress draped with yellow floral blankets and thought to myself,

This is my life now.

I brushed my teeth and changed into pajamas, curling under the stale layers of my new bed. I reflected on the past 48 hours, on flying out of Seattle after a pit-stop to see a friend. On how that friend and I dropped acid and stayed up for the sunrise, omitting sleep and heading straight to my morning flight after a weekend of drinking and doing drugs that don't show up on a urine test. This warped sensation post hallucination distorted reality, sure. The sleep deprivation didn't help, either. But the separation became all too sobering. I looked out my little window by my little bed and told myself:

That was the old me. The hippy, dippy, reckless me.

Just before I drifted into a much-needed sleep I wondered,

Then who am I now?

...

All cozied up in my bed, I slept leisurely without an alarm, waking up at 6am. *Damn jet lag.* The morning sun illuminated my neighborhood through a mildly opaque window, through which I noticed a forest behind my apartment. I grabbed my earphones and headed towards the trees.

This is the new me. I thought.

6am hikes through my backyard trail. This is how 2016 Jenny shows the fuck up.

The air was crisp, with frost glistening on the probing shards of grass. Spring was near and it was welcoming me home. I climbed up the forest of barren maple trees and browning pine, drinking in the morning mist. With the help of my downloaded playlist, I bumped my head to mellow beats and watched the sunshine show promise of warmer days ahead.

I came to a stopping point, or rather a perfectly angled portrait moment to snap for Instagram. I set my phone down and tapped on the self-timer to shoot myself looking off into the distance, all profound and independent, showing off to my followers that I had indeed made it.

Publish.

Refresh

@thatguyjohnnie commented: "Fucking badass"

A rush of praise washed over me. It could have been an after-drip from the LSD. But unlike the acid, this hit was not long-lasting.

...

Be it teammates, roommates, cabinmates or my family - I had always lived with people sharing a common interest. But Korea was the first time I was truly alone. Alone in the home, and due to the language barrier at school, alone in the workplace as well. I chose this solitude to build character. This cultural challenge would prove that I was self-reliant and independent. However, I wasn't so sure if this was all true, and I definitely wasn't sure who I was trying to prove this to.

Was it to my parents, who wanted their college-educated daughter to achieve a well-respected job that they could flaunt to their golf league? Or was it to my former teammates and classmates, knowing they would see my adventurous life from their stale cubicle? Partially, I admit that I wanted to defy societal norms by avoiding car payments, property loans, getting married and having kids. My feminine birthright meant so much more than bearing children; I had come a long way from my high school dream of obtaining an MRS degree in college. I was beginning to understand my privilege as an educated white woman born of an affluent American family, yet I wanted to flee to a place where my privilege would be tested. And while I had every reason to be as happy and free as I portrayed myself online, I bypassed the search for peace and chased validation instead.

Tess met me at my apartment Wednesday morning, leading me to the bus stop for our ride to work. Tess didn't say much, humming and hawing at my eagerness to make a good first impression on the students.

"How is their English? Are they reading yet? Or are we still on the ABCs?" I asked as Tess hit a button to stop the bus. It was such a short ride. *Why didn't we just walk?*

Tess rolled her eyes up to her curly brown bangs and adjusted the zipper of her large gray peacoat.

"Most of the children have English tutors or English-speaking parents, so they will be able to understand you well. But there are a few students that you'll need to be much more patient with. I'll point them out when we begin class." She said, exhausted.

From the stop, we followed a trail up a hill, leading to the hagwon. The contemporary home laid on a couple of acres of land, with a small swing set to the right of the building, a forest on the left, and a vegetable garden in front, about 50 meters long.

The two story hagwon consisted of four bright bedrooms turned classrooms, filled with pale wooden chairs, low tables, and a desk for the teacher, but no whiteboard in sight. There was a small, open-faced kitchen, an office for Sunny, and a large common space on the first floor with a wall of windows leading up to the second story. Within the wide, open entry room was a fireplace and a small desk for me, placed near the front door.

Two yellow school vans pulled up to the driveway, releasing dozens of munchkins to stream out of their booster seats and through the entrance. A pair of handsome toddlers ran towards me as I waved at my new students. They gasped.

"Ahhh!" They looked at each other, laughing, then looked at me.

"Ahhh!" They pointed at me, still laughing.

"Taejong! Sungho!" Tess hissed.

"Say hello to Jenny Teacher, she just came here from America." Tess said as she softened the volume of her voice, raising the pitch.

"Annyeong, Jenny Teacher!" They yelled before darting away.

"Annyeong! Hello!" I laughed back. Never had I been so delighted to have boys scream, then run away from me. *They were all so darn cute.* I had much to learn about classroom management, sure, but seeing these gentle, innocent faces made any rowdiness much more tolerable.

"Tess, where's the curriculum?" I asked with half an hour to spare before the first English class. Tess brought a smile to her face, the first one I'd seen all day.

"There is none," she said.

"What do you mean? How do you make your lesson plans?" I asked, perplexed.

"So..." Tess pulled out four thin workbooks from the stubby white bookcase next to my desk. "You'll ask Sunny to order a new set of books every six months. They will be on level 5 in July, so you'll order those books by June."

"Ok, so we just teach from the book? *This* tiny thing? For six months?" My heart began to pound. *This is all I get to work with?*

"Yes. You'll want to utilize about one page per class." She said, relieved that this work would soon no longer be hers to bear.

"One page for a half-hour class? And the rest of the time... we what, sing the ABCs?" I teased.

"Yea. The kids love "Old Macdonald" Tess said smugly.

"We must go now, it's time for class." Tess grabbed a workbook and led me upstairs to a classroom of eight boys and two girls, which was the gender ratio among my other three classes. Twenty ebony eyes steered my way as their Korean teacher, Bora, greeted me with a bow.

"Welcome, Jenny Teacher. The children are so happy to meet you." Bora stood petite in her black pencil skirt and blouse, grinning ear to ear between her pin-straight hair and bangs that framed her smooth, fair face.

"Thank you!" I beamed. Bora's smile was reassuring. I was feeling a little more confident now, but I knew I had much to learn about the art of teaching.

"Good morning!" I shouted.

"Good morning!" Ten tiny mouths shouted back.

"Ask the children how they are," Tess whispered.

"How are you?" I asked the room.

"I'm happy!" one kid yelled.

"I'm sad!" said the other.

"I'm ANGRY!" A boy got out of his seat and started coming for my knees.

"Taejong! Omo!" Bora launched towards Taejong and started cooing him down, uttering something in Korean then directed him back towards his seat. Less than five minutes had gone by, and I stood there paralyzed, unsure of what to do. I stepped to the side, letting Tess lead the way. She slowly depicted an illustration in the workbook of a child breaking another kid's toy, then apologizing. It was a lesson on forgiveness. Tess then went one-by-one with each kid, asking them to repeat after her: "I'm sorry."

After three more 50-minute classes, it was time for lunch. Tess and I helped the quiet, female cook run food to all the classrooms before eating from our metal tins at my desk. My stainless-steel chopsticks clanked between the dividers, pushing around rice and kimchi with frustration. It wouldn't take too many more lunches for me to surrender my sticks and pick up a fork.

After eating side by side in silence, I turned to Tess to ask, "Where's Sunny?" She took another bite of tofu, swallowed, and then responded with her eyes fixated on her food.

"Um, Sunny comes in and out. She runs a couple other businesses, including the Play Cafe, where you will work on Tuesday's and Thursday's." Tess then relaxed back in her chair, with the faintest smile on her face.

That evening, I mustered enough energy to scope out a gym down the street from my apartment, which offered spin and yoga classes for a low monthly rate. Behind the front desk, dozens of adults all sweat in matching outfits. It was standard to work out in the provided black tees and loose, gray shorts, both branded in the gym's logo. I found this strange until I found it quite convenient, as the laundry service helped me to minimize worry about what I was wearing to my work out. After I signed a 12-month contract, I thanked the front desk clerk for his translation and decided to start exercising *tomorrow*. I stopped at a 7-11 on my walk home, eating onigiri, a sticky rice ball wrapped in seaweed, before I made it to my door. I slipped off my shoes, threw my coat to the ground, and collapsed on my bed. This new routine would involve very little rinse, and a vicious cycle of repeat.

The next day after a full agenda of singing, dancing, and coloring with the children, it was 3pm and time for my two-hour "shift" at the Play Café. Tess led me down a path from the hagwon towards a modern glass building at the bottom of the hill. This cafe sold overpriced coffee, hot Korean snack foods and a hefty entrance fee into a padded playground equipped with slides, rock walls and ball pits.

"What are we supposed to do here?" I asked Tess.

"*You* are supposed to play with the children." She smirked.

"Ok, clear this up for me. On Monday, Wednesday, and Friday, I'll teach until 5:30. But on Tuesday and Thursday I teach until 3 then head here for two hours? To *play* with random children?" I said in frustration, as none of this was mentioned in my teaching contract.

"Yes," Tess nodded.

It wasn't that *playing* with the young children was difficult, more so these children traveled across the suburbs to play with their toddler friends or spend time with their parents who had taken off work, not to be harassed by a random white girl. Most of the kids who came through the cafe were under the age of three as it is common for kids any older to run straight to a tutoring session after school. To my dismay, nearly every time I worked at the Play Cafe, I made a kid cry.

"So sorry" their mom would say.

"Soojin has never seen a foreigner before."

After these rejections from the toddlers, I'd smile at the mom and retreat to the ball pit to drown in desolation.

Once I got into the groove of lesson planning and learning the names of my students, it didn't take long for me to find friends, or at least drinking buddies to party with on the weekends. Thanks to Facebook groups, I locked down prospects for mingling the moment I landed in Incheon. The first acquaintances I met in Seoul were kind and welcoming, yet something about drinking with strangers this time around heightened the loneliness I felt inside. This could have been caused in part by my Irish exits I devised for late-night, liquor-induced binges. Or it could have been the soju.

Soju is a strange variation of distilled rice liquor that was first described to me as "vodka giving up." Traditionally, it is served cold via ceramic containers by the senior of a family or a company, then thrown back for hours until that same senior passes out or reaches for their wallet to pay. Alternatively, for me, soju was sipped from a green plastic bottle and chased down by Coke. I experienced both customs during my time in Korea, but preferred the latter.

During my first few weekends in Seoul, my drinking buddies introduced me to hiking groups, which quickly became my new outlet for meeting people and avoiding isolation. Every weekend, the Seoul Hiking Club would bus foreigners and Koreans alike from the metropolitan area to various corners of the country and lodge us a pension hotel, or a large guesthouse with sleeping mats between a full day of tours. Such tours were affordable, organized, and accommodating to a teacher's schedule.

Perfect. I thought. This was absolutely perfect. I would hike and lose weight. I would spend money on adventure, rather than food. I would surround myself with new friends, rather stow away in privacy and commit a binge. These hiking trips would be *transformational!* And above all, insurance to protect myself *from myself.*

My first trip was to Seoraksan National Park, an UNESCO site known for its granite rock formations drizzled in greenery. Boarding our bus, I asked to sit down next to a curly haired woman with a long, narrow face. Her name was Selena, and she happily complied with my request.

Selena grew up in Cape Town, South Africa, granting her that delicate accent which made me feel nurtured and accepted. I, on the other hand, spoke through a worn mouth that was happy to get a break from the bi-weekly binging and purging I was averaging in that first month. But no binging on this trip - I'd have to hide my crazy until the end of the weekend.

Starting our trek at 4am, our tour group lined outside the bus facing a wall of blackness that was the trailhead. Then two, then three, then six or so lights appeared from the heads of our Korean compadres. Selena and I laughed at our noob status, wearing sneakers and cotton leggings as Koreans in their sixties blazed past us in head lamps, hiking boots and trekking poles. Our laughter turned into heaving breathing as we ascended quickly up the incline. The trail's energy propelled us up the mountain like an uphill stream, synchronizing with the eager pace of fellow hikers striving to reach the summit by sunrise. Selena and I patiently took water breaks with one another, offering words of encouragement between switchbacks.

"Come on, Jenny! Let's beat the sun!" Selena cheered.

And beat it, we did. Upon the summit, a layer of orange divided the vast blue sky into two. Soon, the sun started to rise over Seoraksan, a horizon of jagged rock formations blanketed in emerald shrubs. One by one, the clouds came out. Selena and I sat for about half an hour in thin air, catching our breath and commencing our newfound friendship.

"Wow. It's quite magnificent, isn't it?" Selena smiled at me.

"Shall we take a photo?" She asked.

Flattered that someone wanted to be seen with me, I reached for my phone and opened the camera. My cheeks bore extra padding to them from just one month in Korea, but I stretched them wide anyways as Selena and I snapped a selfie among the mountains.

The hike down was just as magnificent, on a path of granite stacked tall and serrated. With two hours left in our descent, Selena and I found a smooth surface of rock to lay down on and stretch.

"Jenny, I'm so glad I had you for motivation. You were my coach up there!" Selena said as we laid beneath the sun.

"Likewise." I hesitated, stuck with stiffness. What did Selena see in me? Couldn't she tell I was suffering? Should I *tell* her I was in deep, existential pain? No, no. Better to save face than scare my new friend away…

While these weekend getaways suspended binges through social restraints, the wrath returned tenfold once I reached my apartment. No matter the time of day, my quiet street provided snacks around the clock. I had five cafes to choose from on my walk to work for carbs and caffeine, dozens of 24-hour stores to visit at my convenience, and a couple late-night chimaek spots.

Chimaek, or Chikin and Maekju (beer), is offered in finer dine-in restaurants, walk up to-go windows, gas stations and street markets. Locals and expats can sip cheap lager and chew on this fried delicacy at any time, from park picnics to BYO chimaek at baseball games. I, however, devoured these glazed nuggets by the bucket in the comfort of my shoebox apartment, so that the toilet was only a few feet away. As tasty as Korean chicken was, it was not cheap or easy to upchuck, but I'd manage to scrape up some Korean Won after a purge, then rinse and repeat at a different vendor.

The question was never *if* I would binge, but how soon and on what foods. The desire to devour usually began between lunch and my walk home, when I would decide whether I would wait until after the gym or turn the entire night into a wash.

Am I going to be "good" today and make it to spin class? Or will I start eating on my walk home from school?

On "bad" days, the verdict to eat materialized the moment I woke up. There was no reasoning with my disease. I was bound to binge.

This is how it's going to be, Jen. You'll hop into the bakery chain for a milk bun, a potato pancake, and a bottled latte. At school, it's Yoo-Jin's birthday, where you'll be offered plenty of cake and chocolate. For lunch, you will per usual eat a second serving of rice and that crack sauce they call gochujang, then sneak into Yoo-Jin's classroom while the children are taking violin lessons to check for leftover cake. On your walk home, you'll stop by the local bakery for sugar-covered hot dogs wrapped in pretzel buns. And don't forget their chocolate croissants. The bakery with the bear on the logo has the best croissants.

When you're ready to throw up, go to 7/11 for ice cream and milk, to help the purge come up easier. If that's not enough, you still have rice and sweet potatoes in the fridge you so diligently meal prepped the other night. How's that diet going for you, anyway?

Most days, it was much easier to give into the disease, as long as I had enough money to feed it. Other days, I walked to school without my wallet to avoid spending on the way home or would head straight to my gym to delay the binge. On the occasions I did not carry my backpack to school, I extended my walk home to a two-hour stroll on a trail through the city, weaving around rivers and outdoor gyms. This gentle exercise was all I could handle most afternoons, as I was often strung out from sugar. I listened to old playlists while passing hundreds of Koreans on the trail, imagining myself back in America at the concerts of my favorite artists. I reminisced on summer shows and music festivals, knowing that I wouldn't be able to enjoy smoking and swaying to indie rock among a crowd of skinny girls in crop tops looking the way I did. It was best if I stayed safe by living thousands of miles away. I was already an outcast, foreign and overweight. I was already in the perfect place to hide in shame.

By summertime, I was fat, broke, and far from happy. Besides food, my paychecks mostly went towards hiking tours. I thought I was clever to spend my money immediately after each paycheck, permitting a small budget for food with the remaining balance. Though I wasn't balancing *anything* in Korea. A lack of funds didn't stop me from foraging. I'd steal packaged cookies here and there, and never at the same shops. It was easy to steal in the subway markets, swiping candy bars during the heavy flow of rush hour commutes. Nights before payday, I'd splurge on a chimaek dinner, zeroing out my account to buy a family-sized meal, eating for one. I'd wake up penniless, relieved that I did not have the means to binge until Friday. Then the voices would return, enticing me to grab my credit card and rack up high interest debt on food I would waste, manipulating my meals in sick and twisted ways.

Come payday, I'd take out cash as my two-week allotment, then drop my debit card into a cup of water, storing it into my mini fridge's ice bin. The idea was to suspend eating frenzies by literally freezing my funds. Sure,

205

this tactic prolonged the compulsion, but it only angered the insatiable entity inside. Ed, my eating disorder, was now possessed by disease. And that disease consumed me.

If I wasn't spending money on booze, food, or excursions, I dropped a considerable amount on face masks, because, you know, *self-care*. Beauty stores were ubiquitous throughout Seoul, with plastic surgeon advertisements plastered along every bus and subway corridor. Whenever I visited the affluent neighborhood of Gangnam, I invariably passed women with bandages on their noses and bruises under their eyes. But the procedures didn't stop there. I soon found out that Korea hosted the most plastic surgeries per capita *in the world*, with people going under the knife for chin and forehead augmentations, the popular double-eyelid fold, and of course, hella lip injections and Botox. An ignorant statement that I would hear before my move was that "all Asians look alike." Though I was starting to see some truth to this stereotype, as people all around me were throwing time and money into overnight clinics where they could transform their face and come out looking like their favorite K-Pop star.

Now I'll admit, I saved a few K-pop songs to my playlists and got a rise watching their trippy music videos while running from a treadmill at my gym. Though soon after, I'd head home to eat and numb out on Netflix. I flew through television seasons, watching anything from *Suits* to *Narcos* until 2am. This sedentary habit paired well with my binging, as TV was the only thing I had energy for on a bloated stomach and a head full of sugar. When a 45-minute episode required too much focus for my monkey mind, I turned to YouTube to watch vloggers in Los Angeles and New York roll around on hoverboards while filming their day between matcha lattes and outdoor workouts.

That's what I want to be when I grow up.

Their lives seemed so effortless as I watched, awestruck.

I want to inspire others to live the life of their dreams by filming my own.

By now, my Instagram feed was filled with mountain ranges and exotic markets, drenched in commentary from followers "wanting my life." I had built a brand based on travel motivation, but behind the camera I buried myself in deceit. Teaching and travel were supposed to bring me meaning, but the core of my motives was driven by disease. I now lived by the "ABC's" both in and out of the classroom: *Always **Be** Consuming.*

It'd be a stretch to say that I *loved* teaching, however, those little nuggets became my daily bundle of joy. Their round, smiling faces and opaque eyes depended on me for guidance. For leadership. Or at least, for entertainment. Teaching is a selfless profession anywhere in the world and in Korea, considered a well-respected occupation. Though as a foreigner, any praise I might have received was often overshadowed by my Korean colleagues. This cultural hierarchy should have humbled me, and yet, my hunger to be seen only increased.

Come late summer, I booked a last-minute escape to the Jinju Lantern Festival, located in a seaport city at the tip of the Korean peninsula. Expecting copious likes on photos of neon lights, I almost didn't go. I passed out in a binging spell the night before, missing my alarm and the tour bus the next morning. Frantic at the bus terminal, I hurriedly texted Sue, my Korean friend who invited me to the weekend excursion and carefully detailed how I could meet her across the country using public transportation.

Sue was the first person in Korea who I felt safe sharing the details of my disease with. She studied psychology at UCLA before living in Santa Barbara as a counselor throughout her twenties. This allowed her to hold space for the severity of what I was going through, helping me feel okay about not being okay. As the last time I had disclosed to a drinking buddy the lengths of my binging, the pal responded, "we all overeat from time to time."

But Sue understood that I was overeating *every time*. What she didn't understand, however, was why I labeled my behavior before a proper diagnosis.

"Why do you consider yourself diseased? Do you think that sounds a little harsh?" Sue asked.

"Well..." I second guessed my verbiage. "It's what I've been taught. My dad stays sober by admitting he has a disease, and that seems to work for him. I don't view food the same way as other people do. I obsess over food every day, and that certainly isn't normal. How I eat and how *much* I eat isn't normal. So, labeling this abnormality as a disease makes more sense than wondering what the hell is wrong with me." I told Sue.

"There's nothing wrong with you." She responded.

Then why does it feel like something is missing?

When I arrived in Jinju, I spotted my tall Korean friend outside the GS25 convenience store we planned to meet at and ran up to hug her in relief. Behind Sue stood an even taller, fairer skinned woman dressed in a pink bomber jacket and ripped jeans. The bedazzled blonde shot selfies from a rubber cell phone case resembling a prescription bottle that said, "CHILL PILLS". When she set the phone down, her bright blue eyes beamed at me under her long, platinum hair.

"오모 Omo!" She cried.

"Who is this beauty?!" She held her arms out for a hug, and I stiffened right up, taking a moment to realize she was speaking to me.

A part of me wanted to judge this breathing Barbie doll for littering sparkles, but I couldn't help but stare at her shine. Maybe her ostentatious appearance invigorated my dulled senses. Maybe I thought she was cool. Either way, Ava the Canadian instantly became my most interesting, unlikely, nurturing friend in Korea.

Ava's brazen style seamlessly made her stand out from the crowd. She was colorful, sometimes punk, and always pretty in her detailed nails and bright lipsticks. Her smooth voice and clear skin were unbothered by the number of cigarettes she consumed in a day. Ava ate well and ate often, yet nothing seemed to stick on her long bones. Her decorative dress was much to conspicuous for me to consider, but damn, she rocked it.

That weekend in Jinju, Sue, Ava and I hiked up to an ancient temple on top of a mountain, overlooking a range of dark greenery that was weeks away from turning colors for fall. The late August heat was no match for Ava's makeup, thanks to her trusted pocket fan. As the sun and temperatures dropped, we made our way to the lantern festival - a park of grand illumination. Neon dragons, lotuses, warriors and emperors came to life for the festival, and floated along the reflective ponds. We walked under a blanket of red lanterns to get to a path where patrons could sit and order food by the water under red and green pagodas. Ava and I sat next to each other the entire time, laughing and drinking the night away. Sue didn't seem too fond of my new friendship, as this trip was the last weekend I ever spoke to my counselor companion.

On our ride back to Seoul, the tour bus stopped at a rest station, where a fellowship of Korean Jehovah's Witnesses recruited outside.

"Omo! My parents are Jehovah's Witnesses. I'm going to say hi." Ava darted out the bus to make friendly conversation, while Sue shot an uncomfortable look on her face, avoiding me, Ava, and the fellows at all costs. I followed Ava to the group handing out pamphlets, listened as she spoke Korean then joined her back on the bus.

"People can believe what they want about the church. They are always *so kind*. I know some people think the Jehovah's Witnesses are crazy and radical, but they aren't hurting anyone. It's just one belief system that gets a lot of negative attention, really." Ava commented.

Not knowing much about the JW doctrine myself, I shrugged in agreement. What was I to say? I surely had no direction towards the divine. But I did believe in one thing - that bulimia is a disease, one of which I had

209

undoubtedly. After five months of regular purging, I was starting to get desperate. So, I gave God another chance.

...

When I sat through my first 12-step Overeaters Anonymous meeting in southwest Florida, I left feeling hopeless, caught up in the idea that I'd end up like many of the members: obese. When I washed my mouth off from the vomit of my first purge in Korea, I stared into a pair of empty eyes. The mirror reflected a warning:

Those meetings may seem hopeless, but so is another night of gluttony. You've got nothing to lose, only more weight to gain.

This dread led me to search for OA in Seoul, which held one English meeting on Tuesday nights in the city. The commute would take me an hour by train to make the hour-long meeting, which meant three hours of my Tuesday that I would not spend eating. The train rides to and from, however, started to get in the way of this thinking.

I'll eat two milk buns during the ride, stopping for one of those waffles with whipped cream at Yaksu station. But this time *will be the* last time*. This meeting I'll mean it. I'll stop. Things will be different.*

Our church basement meetings included the same four women: a Czech girl studying at Seoul University, a Korean American from Boston, a Korean woman who spoke broken English, and my first sponsor, Beth, who was an army wife living off the U.S. base in a popular expatriate neighborhood called Itaewon.

Beth had been "abstinent" for nearly six months and was a sponsee of the Bostonian woman. Her abstinence consisted of three meals a day, nothing in between. Beth logged and submitted her food to her sponsor each night via call, text, or email. With grit and the higher power she called God, Beth achieved abstinence from compulsive overeating.

Abstinence with drugs and alcohol is black and white. It's complete avoidance. It's in no way easy, but it's a clear line. As for food addiction, the line blurs into gray matter, because someone's "safe" food of say, peaches, could be another person's crack. My drug of choice was anything creamy, salty, sweet, or processed, and I would go any length to grab my bag. Sometimes the itch started in the middle of the night, where I'd run to my dealer, the clerk at 7-11, for honey-laced potato chips and eat them in my bed. I was perpetually strung out on sugar, plotting my next chance to re-up and throw up.

I desperately wished I had something stronger and less humiliating than cinnamon twists to overdose on. But unlike drugs, alcohol, porn or impulsive shopping, my vice: a gluttonous and deadly sin, was not one I could abstain from. My dad had to quit drinking altogether to change his life around. But I had to eat to live, even though I was slowly killing myself with food every day.

I had long ago lost the primitive instincts of hunger cues. Between sporadic fasting and continuous meals, my body assumed a state of incessant appetite. Every binge got bigger, its cycle lasting longer, and starting earlier each day.

I told myself: *You're disgusting, Jenny. Last night was despicable. You ate an entire pizza with breadsticks. And when that wasn't enough, you threw it up to make room for half a quart of ice cream before you washed that down the kitchen sink. You should be five dress sizes larger than you are. You should be 300 pounds. You may be able to hide your belly bloat under a sweatshirt and yoga pants, but you know where your fate lies: fat and alone.*

Bullied by my brain, I sought out sanity in OA, hoping the message would lubricate the strident sounds of my mind's grinding gears. My obtrusive thoughts were subdued during meetings, but they came back with vengeance. As I listened to Beth speak on her path of recovery, I could hear my disease gossiping about me from outside the church doors.

This is useless. YOU are useless. Just like your attempt to exercise yesterday.

Beth's story of growing up as the fat kid then sneaking around her husband and kids to eat as an adult did not quite resonate for me as a single twenty-three-year-old who spent my childhood in sports. It was Beth's ability to *stop* overeating which piqued my interest, as she had abstained six months without a binge, whereas I couldn't count the last time I went six *days* without giving into gluttony.

While Beth was a mom, a Christian, and identified as someone who had always been overweight, we shared the same visceral desire to overeat. The principal in picking a sponsor is to "find someone who has what you want." Though I never imagined myself as an army wife in Itaewon, I was willing to do almost anything to obtain six months of normal eating under my belt.

Think of how much weight you will lose by simply *not* binging! After six months of normal portions, you're sure to slim down to a size 4. Then, once you've been able to eat like a decent human again, you can start to restrict again, and will finally fit into the dresses from college waiting for you in your closet back home.

I asked Beth to be my sponsor with the end goal in mind = *weight loss*. For this reason, I was dedicated. I was desperate. I was willing to follow her direction, determined to be the best sponsee that Seoul had ever seen.

As a caregiver, Beth could sugarcoat any dire situation with a smile and a nervous laugh. She was a bit startled by my request but happily sponsored me, as this position would ideally strengthen her own recovery. Beth hammered out mottos passed down from her Bostonian sponsor, including "one day at a time," and "work the steps and watch it work."

The women in our OA meetings had followed the same guideline. Using a food scale, we would weigh out our portions of food for the next day, rationing "points" for proteins, fats, starches, and vegetables. Fruits were a rarity, and sugar was prohibited. Below is a copy of an email I sent to Beth regarding my POE, or *Plan of Eating:*

Breakfast:

2 HB eggs

1 medium banana (I can weigh after I peel it in the morning if you think it's necessary)

25g mixed nuts.

Lunch:

2HB eggs

230 g Broccoli

230 g peppers

100 g rice

Dinner:

100g chicken

230g carrots

230g lettuce

25g dressing

The first day of devoting myself to the meal plan, I was on fire.

This is too easy! I've got a diet and an accountability partner to help me stick to it. There's no need to overeat when you've already got your food laid out for you, that is, unless... wait, is that? No... Is that an extra 30 grams of broccoli you have left in the fridge? You can't possibly let that produce go to waste. Why would Beth care if you ate extra broccoli*? There's no such thing as binging on vegetables. That is, unless, there is. Which means... no! You've overeaten. You've gone over your meal plan by 30 grams of cruciferous veggies. You're a failure. Might as well eat the foods you really want to, throw it up, and try again tomorrow.*

After the binge, I had to decide between lying about my eating or admitting my wrongs. I opted to disclose what had happened. Luckily, Beth was both understanding and patient with me, rooting me on each time I reported a new meal plan and jumped back on the steps. For every day I ate in "abstinence," my disease hung out in the bakeries, waiting to strike at any moment of weakness. And weak I became, feeling so deprived from the sugar I was addicted to. My relapses increased in intensity, forcing me to turn back to Beth, in fear that the program was making my problem worse.

"Use the tools, Jenny. They work when you work them." She told me kindly. Though after a few days, I fell back into the food. One morning after a binge and purge, I picked up my phone to dial someone outside of OA. I needed to confide in the person who brought me into the world with an insatiable genetic code. I called my dad for the first time in months, as I rarely reached out to my family during this isolating year.

"Dad...." I answered, my voice already shaking.

"Hey, hun. How are you?" He said, sounding as steady as ever.

"I'm... I'm not well. My eating... is out of control. I've been going to meetings in the city, but after every string of controlled eating, I relapse harder and longer." I took a pause, hoping his answer to my next question would soothe my erratic thoughts.

"When you got sober, did you ever relapse?"

Please, say yes, Dad. Please tell me you tried, failed, and tried again over and over like I have, then tell me how you overcame your addiction.

"No, Jenny. But I didn't really have a choice. After my second DUI, I was sentenced to AA, and at the time, all my drinking buddies mocked me, saying, 'Martin, you'll never make it.' I was too stubborn to let them watch me fail."

My heart dropped into my rumbling stomach. I was his kin, we shared the same genetic makeup. And despite how stubborn I was, my steadfast attitudes were no match for my eating. My disease made me feel delusional and disconnected from everyone, including my family.

"But Jenny, drugs and drinking are so different. You don't need them to live. I don't fully understand what you're going through, but you must have grace. You can't just quit food."

When we hung up, I cried for an hour as I walked around aimlessly. As much as I loved him, I couldn't turn to my dad for guidance around food. And so, I turned to the tools, hoping to fix what felt irreversibly broken:

A Plan of Eating

Been there, done that. I come from a restrictive background of eating egg whites between two-hour swim practices, and now I'm told to weigh out my broccoli? That's whack. *Next.*

Sponsorship

Beth is my sponsor because she has what I want: six months of well-portioned meals. *Cool, next.*

Meetings

I've got Tuesday nights down, but the Big Book asks us to go as much as possible. I tried telephone meetings, but those suckers on the other line have no idea if I'm eating during the call or not. Besides, I'm not obligated to pay attention, or at least pretend to pay attention on the phone like I am during a face-to-face meeting. *What else you got?*

Telephone

Pick up the phone before you pick up the food. That's easy enough when you can trick anyone into thinking that everything is ok. I may not be able to hide the bloat in my cheeks after a purge, but I can sure as hell prep my voice to act as if all is well and going according to (my food) plan.

Writing

I've been journaling for years, filling each page with "Be healthier", "Work out more", "Lose 10 pounds by March" and "NO GLUTEN,

NO DAIRY, NO SUGAR". Though since starting the program, my entries looked like so:

Day 1 - *easy peasy, you got this.*

Day 2 - *Make it another day*

Day 3 - *I can and I will!*

Day 4 - *I forgive myself from my wrong doings and surrender to God in temptation for the future*

Day 9 - *Be humble, warrior*

Day 1 - *Fresh day, fresh start. Make this one count!*

Day 1 - *I give my power to God to help me restore my sanity from relapse*

Day 2 - *I am enough. I have enough. I do enough. Jenny - no binging*

Day 1 - *I am powerless over food, and my life has become unmanageable*

Day 1 - *My disease plays me like a string puppet, pulling me towards the bakery. It is a demon weighing me down, screaming for attention and for the food. Through God, I may ask for Him to cut these strings so I may walk in my own will, consequently flicking off the devil that hangs by my side. I will soon wear tank tops, to look left and right and see nothing but toned shoulders. Then I will look up. Not to see ED in control as the puppet master, but to see the clear blue sky God has graced me with.*

Literature

Reading isn't really my thing, as I've got a long list of Netflix originals to catch up on. OA podcasts, however, I can manage. Listening to recovery stories through my earphones is like sitting in a meeting and making a phone call. *Three birds, one stone.*

I carried these tools around like armor, protecting me from myself. One tool that wasn't listed in the OA website but was mentioned in every meeting was prayer - to God - as if begging to some elusive entity would relieve me from my madness.

"Ask God to remove your cravings," Beth would suggest. But that seemed so... simple. Surely, drinking water would be a better appetite suppressant.

But I was desperate, so I tried. I got on my knees in the mornings, sighed and said:

"God, help me to not be crazy today."

And though I didn't exactly believe that anyone was listening, my hands weren't picking up food when they were pressed together. Praying soon became the only time I found myself kneeling for something other than the toilet.

By September, I was binging three to four times a week. One afternoon, I was on the third consecutive day of an eating spell, and I had depleted every resource from my tool kit. I walked home from school with the OA podcasts playing in my ear, reminding me that *the program works when you work it*. But something else played louder in my head, which was the demand for a milk bun. Those plump, gooey blobs of dough baked just enough to fill with sweet cream softened the inside of my dry mouth the moment I would take a bite. The 1,000 won milk bun cost me less than one American dollar to buy and met every criterion of a proper binge food: processed with flour and sugar and easy to throw back up.

To ease my cravings, I called Beth and the three other women in my program. No answers. I dropped my wallet in my apartment and decided to walk off this urge, heading towards the trail with a couple of OA episodes cued. On the podcast, a woman in her fifties spoke of her sixteen-year abstinence after numerous relapses, but all I could hear was the plea for that goddamn milk bun.

Once I hit the trail head, I pulled out my earphones and ran straight to the river. Between the pavement and the water was a thick plane of tall grass, tall enough to hide a frantic woman in despair. The podcasts didn't seem to work. My phone calls went to voicemail, but I knew I had one more tool to turn to. I fell to my knees and prayed by the river, asking God to take away my ridiculous obsession around this stupid milk bun.

I kneeled for minutes, crying into my empty hands.

God, help me please!

I murmured under my breath, hoping my voice could trump the noise in my head.

God, I'm here. Are you?

I longed for a bolt of lightning to pierce through my soul, to burn through the faulty wires in my brain and save me from spending money at the bakery. Eventually, my panicked breath began to slow down, allowing me to hear the calming winds on the water. With ten million Koreans in Seoul, I searched up and down the river without spotting another human. I was alone and god was nowhere to be found.

I treaded back to my apartment in silence, set my phone down with resentment and immediately retrieved my wallet for five thousand won. My heart beat louder as I neared the bakery chain that sold the milk buns, and I took a deep breath like someone preparing to knock on a door before greeting their date. But instead of the first-date jitters, I was plagued by a grim uneasiness. After all that praying, I found myself back at the bakery. So much for a higher power.

I tried everything, yet I'm still yearning to eat. If god is real, then who is in control?

I opened the doors and nodded at the employees who nodded back at their best customer. With won in my pocket, I had no intention to steal. Though something made me feel like I already committed a sinister act. I was ridden in guilt, sensing that someone other than the staff was watching over me.

God, is that you watching over my shoulder? I still have time to walk out. If you are real, I'll leave. If not, I'll…

Wait! What the?!

No milk buns!!! No FLIPPING milk buns? I went through all that hell by the river and now no milk buns?

Ugh, fine. I'll buy chocolate.

Whether god was present or as absent as the milk buns, one thing was certain. My disease had won. And unlike the milk buns, my disease wasn't going anywhere.

By October, I slipped into a week-long spiral of uncontrollable purging. It started one Saturday morning after a black-out, where I wrote in my journal "No dairy or gluten!" which resulted in me binging on exactly those ingredients (think: milk bun). I threw up every day for a week straight, waking up every morning with the thought; "I'm alive!" before realizing, "I did it again last night, didn't I?" My eyes would then focus on the empty food containers collecting in the corner of my apartment. I stared back up to the ceiling to ask myself, "Will this day be any different?"

This trance followed me to school, where I stole snacks whenever there was a surplus. On a Wednesday, I was eating at my desk and smacked a mosquito biting my inner thigh, which had me itching my legs hours into the night. The next day, a rash emerged. I gave it a scratch but didn't think much of it as I dressed. But the itching persisted, and by my last class on Friday afternoon, I lifted my shirt to reveal the red, blotchy skin now spreading onto my stomach.

"Jenny teacher dirty!" One child laughed.

"Jenny teacher no shower!" Another added.

Sadly, the kids were right. I hadn't showered and was dripping in my own filth. I immediately imagined the candy wrappers piling up in my apartment and the smell of vomit in my bathroom. I pressed my tongue to my teeth to imagine the decay imposing through my enamel, wondering if the kids could sense any other impurities.

One of the Korean teachers turned to me and gasped,

"Food allergy!"

The thought hadn't hit me before, but now it made sense. *Dairy and gluten!*

A hope that I could possibly be dairy and/or gluten intolerant left me optimistic on my walk home. *God, please make me celiac! All those gluten free bitches are so skinny. I'd do anything to have a real, diagnosed allergy to this god-forbidden grain. And with no dairy, no chocolate. No ice cream. No milk buns. Everything I binge on contains dairy or gluten. I may finally get my break.*

The rash on my inner thigh spread further, reaching around to my butt and up to my belly button. What I initially thought was a mosquito bite was now potentially a food allergy, which I desperately hoped was the case. This could be my cure! As being allergic to my binge foods would inhibit my ability to eat them… so I told myself.

What followed was an idea I can only describe as utter insanity. I developed a hypothesis that if I took antihistamines while binging on dairy and gluten, then one of two results would arise:

1- The rash persisted, meaning I was for sure intolerant to my favorite binge foods, or

2- The rash cleared up, meaning the drugs worked and I should buy some bug spray.

I woke up Saturday with the same amount of redness, but now the blotches had hardened. Still testing my scientific study, I bought hydrocortisone cream and stronger antihistamine. At least that's what I think I bought when I went to the pharmacy and lifted up my shirt, watched the pharmacist stare in horror, and offer me a cream and some drugs to help heal my rash.

I canceled my weekend beach plans to celebrate a friend's birthday, secretly thankful that this rash provided an excuse to avoid swimsuits and socializing. Instead of sun, I cruised through another season of *Jane the Virgin* while gnawing on 20 pieces of fried chicken. After this week of continuous purging, however, I was too exhausted to expel my food and figured it was best I keep whatever the pharmacist had prescribed down in my system. The only time I left my apartment on Sunday was to buy ramen and cookies at the 7-11 next to my building, as any further would be too taxing. It finally dawned on me that this rash was certainly hives, and whatever I had done to cause such an outbreak was only worsening. If I was truly allergic to dairy and gluten, then at least I'd have a reason to give up so many of the foods I had manipulated for years. But the question was: *Was I willing to abstain today for the sake of saving my life?*

The answer was no, and I went back to the store to shove down and throw up ice cream.

Waking up on Monday, I felt hungover, yet I hadn't drunk in a week. My eyes felt heavy, despite wasting the weekend in bed. I peeled off my blanket and stared down at my legs.

O shit!

The hives had spread down to my calves and reached up towards my arms and elbows. Pushing my body out of bed took more energy than I anticipated, leaving me dizzy as I sat up. The hives pulled tight on my skin, burning with ferocity.

I tiptoed into the bathroom, aching all over. I caught a glimpse of Medusa in the mirror and froze to stone.

Ohhh sheeeeet.

I was oddly stoic. I did not panic. I did not cry. I *couldn't* cry, considering my eye lids, lips and ears looked like a toddler took a filler needle to my face and aggressively stabbed with abandon.

I sent photos of my swollen, pink face to my mom, hoping she would tell me what to ask for at the pharmacy and that I was going to be ok. Too disassociated from my body, I was unable to assess the severity of this breakout. Besides, I was running late for work.

I was afraid Sunny would reprimand me for calling off sick for work, so I decided to show the teachers my condition before the students arrived. God forbid my facial deformity make a child cry.

"오모 Omo!" Bora screamed, holding her hands to her heart in sympathy.

"Jenny Teacher! Your face! Go, go to hospital!" Bora continued. She ardently agreed to tell Sunny about my absence and directed me to the ER clinic down the road.

I was reluctant to visit the hospital at first, mostly because I feared what they might charge me. But as I caught another reflection of myself, I realized yea, I should go get this shit checked out.

After ten minutes in the waiting room, a steroid shot, and a plethora of antibiotics, I checked out of the emergency room with an 8,000 won bill. In American currency, that's just under eight dollars. Eight *freaking* dollars for an ER visit. Damn, I thought, I should have headed to the doctor's office sooner.

But before I left, the doctor told me one thing. Unfortunately, it wasn't that I was celiac or allergic to dairy. Without any explanation, he advised me to abstain from dairy, meat, and eggs.

Dairy, meat, and eggs. Wait a minute, that's a vegan diet. Did a doctor just shoot me up with steroids for under ten dollars and give me nutritional advice? Who would have thunk, a medical professional attempting to approach healing from an inexpensive, non-invasive, holistic remedy...

By the time I made it to my apartment, I could tell the steroid shot was kicking in. The voice that usually told me to binge was now reciting a different message: *no dairy, no meat, no eggs*. With the day off from work, I decided to take a break from Netflix and do some research. I opened my laptop to YouTube, typed in "Veganism" and slid down a rabbit hole of vloggers and activists, eventually turning me onto a video that left a scar from this harrowing day.

A vegan YouTuber shared her eating disorder recovery story, saying that veganism had helped her eat in abundance without causing harm to herself or other sentient beings. The YouTuber then detailed a story of another woman's eating disorder, who suffered from bulimia. She showed a photo of this bulimic woman after an extended cycle of binging and purging, which caused her to break out in hives all over her body. As the photo of the bulimic woman's rash enlarged in the video, my pupils dilated in distress. I was starting to see myself on the screen.

The YouTuber then somberly announced that the bulimic woman's heart had failed a day after she shot the photos. She was dead. I shut my laptop as a chill ran over my dry, red skin.

I am literally killing myself with bulimia.

And yet, I'm still here.

This video made me realize that my breakout wasn't some sort of allergic reaction, but that my body had gone into bulimic shock. The stoic state I had sustained all day shattered as I screamed into my pillow and sobbed.

God didn't want me to die. God gave me a second chance.

I wish I could say this was the last time I ever purged. I wish I could say that this was a white-light moment, and that I had reached nadir. But as a traveling addict, I frequented rock bottom. This health scare was less of a turning point, and more of a wake-up call that there was a higher power out there, watching over to protect and make sure I stayed alive.

...

After that wake-up call from God, an entity I was starting to believe in, a few things had shifted. Like trying veganism and medication. Key word = tried.

Beth referred me to her psychiatrist in Itaewon who prescribed me Zoloft, an antidepressant, and Klonopin, an anti-anxiety med, within minutes of my arrival in their office. While I was a proponent of recreational drugs, pharmaceuticals had always rubbed me the wrong way. I viewed SSRIs as a band-aid fix for depression, but after my most recent health scare, I thought *what the hell, what else you got to lose?*

After a week of taking Zoloft and eating a plant-based diet, I felt good. *Real good.* My energy was up, my skin was clearing, and while I was still too ashamed to face the scale, I could tell by my waistline that I had lost some weight. Even so, the biggest factor in this mood boost may have been from planning my upcoming trip to Thailand to visit my dear, dear friend, Brooklyn.

Brooklyn moved to Bangkok just a month after I moved to Seoul, and I'd like to think I inspired her to make the leap and teach English abroad. But unlike my year in Asia, Brooklyn was kicking some serious ass. She had traveled across Thailand's infamous islands and hidden gems. She could speak conversational Thai, which came in handy when hailing tuk-tuks. Upon arrival, she led me to her humid apartment to refresh for the night, handing me a 5-gallon jug for my bath, as her building was observing a water ration. While I splashed suds under my breasts and armpits, Brooklyn played an unfamiliar tune from her dresser. It was Tame Impala.

"What is this?" I asked from the tub.

"Keep listening, you'll like it." She smiled as she swayed her hips to "The Less I Know the Better. "

It dawned on me that I hadn't changed up my music in months. The only update I had on popular culture was on Taylor Swift's *Bad Blood* video people kept posting on Facebook. I had been living under a rock, or better put, with my head in porcelain.

Once bathed, I followed Brooklyn around the noisy streets of her neighborhood. From a bus stop, we piled into the bed of a large red truck, sliding down the wood panel seats shaped in a "U." I popped my head out of the windows of the makeshift roof, watching smoke rise from traffic. Buses, motorbikes, and trucks funneled their way through the streets, hardly following road signs and traffic lights. A tuk-tuk came straight at us, weaving through a wave of vehicles. I shot a terrified and dramatic look at Brooklyn.

"This is where we *die!*" I whispered.

"There, there. We'll be ok. I take this ride nearly every day." Brooklyn giggled.

We made it to our stop alive, despite the number of red lights the driver ran. A diamond mesh fence gated the entrance to the night market, opening to a field of vendors separated by hanging tarp, draped in string lights. We passed exotic fruit stands of coconut, mango, lychee, and the controversial durian, known as "stinky fruit." The spiky exterior of this football-shaped food takes a sharp knife, and sometimes the help of a hammer to retrieve the yellow meat inside. Intrigued, I bought a bowl of the sour-smelling fruit and followed Brooklyn down to a corner of cooks preparing vegetable Pad Thai. Brooklyn bought us a heaping plate of noodles and headed to the picnic tables where we ate among hundreds of people under red tents. As I picked at my sweet and savory durian fruit, my eyes widened while taking my first bite into this oddly creamy texture, tasting a bit like caramelized garlic. *I loved it.*

"What do you think, Jen?" Brooklyn asked.

"Well... I like everything and this isn't too bad!" I said. "Though I will let you know, I'm vegan now. It's only been a couple weeks, but I already feel so good. Besides, not buying meat has saved me a lot on groceries."

"O wow. Good for you!" Brooklyn cheered.

"I can't say the same. I eat meat every day. I also eat out every day. It's cheaper than buying groceries. But all the oil from street food has made me put on some weight." Brooklyn stared down on her stomach that seemed slightly softer than the last time I'd seen her.

Weight gain in Asia? Tell me about it…

I bragged on about my veganism until Brooklyn stopped me to ask, "what about shrimp?"

"What about shrimp? It's seafood, so it's not vegan." I responded.

She pointed at my noodles and sighed, "Sorry girl, but the Thai put shrimp in everything. See those little crunchy things? That's shrimp. I'll try ordering for you next time, but fish and meat are so ingrained in their cuisine. I wouldn't be surprised if most of the broth we'll eat this weekend is made from beef."

Well hot damn! So much for veganism!

This news left me a little bummed but forced me to be gracious with myself. If I couldn't eat vegan, I could at least enjoy what I was eating. I had traveled this far to see Brooklyn in a country which was so high on my bucket list, that I wasn't going to dampen my experience by whining over my arbitrary dietary restrictions. I witnessed first-hand the care the Thai people put into their meals as they prepared their food, delivering our plates with great pride. Why strip that joy away because I had watched *Cowspiracy* half a dozen times?

The next morning, Brooklyn and I packed our weekend bags for a getaway to Koh Chang, an unspoiled island of jungles and luscious mountains, on the eastern edge of the Gulf of Thailand. A tuk tuk, a train, a flight and boat ride later, Brooklyn and I arrived at our quiet resort. While my teacher's salary could hardly afford my eating habits in Korea, Brooklyn and I were able to split a beachside bungalow for about twenty USD each a night in Thailand. After a couple minutes of oo-ing and ah-ing at our little hut with a bamboo porch and a palm thatched roof, we dressed up for a night out.

After a hot shower, Brooklyn and I hit the small township in Koh Chang. Dimly lit bars and small hotels lined the dirt road we walked along, while motorcycles buzzed past us as we scanned for a place to drink. As the sun set, we popped our heads through a couple of hostel bars, settling on one Brooklyn picked for its pool tables. We headed up to a tiki hut and ordered mojitos when Brooklyn grabbed hold of my shoulder as she stood in shock.

"What?" I asked.

"I *know* that guy." She got all giddy, the way she does around a crush. I followed her gaze towards the pool table to a tan, muscular man with a baby face and thick, dark hair.

"What do you mean you *know* that guy? We're on an island in Thailand. How cou-"

"We matched on Tinder when I was in Pattaya! His name is Bastien. He's French."

I tried to keep my eyes from rolling.

"Ah, of course you know Bastien from France here on an island in Thailand." I sighed.

"I gotta talk to him." And just like that, deja vu from the magic spas in Budapest seeped through my straw. I started double fisting both of our mojitos while Brooklyn bent backwards for Bastien from France. When both glasses hollowed out, I concluded my conversation with the bartender and made way towards Brooklyn, who was playing pool with her Tinder match.

"Oh! Jenny!" She smiled.

Yes, it's me, your friend who traveled all the way from Korea to spend time with you.

Brooklyn whispered in my ear, "Bastien has a coworker we can set you up with. He's over at the other bar. His name is Sean."

Flashbacks of the magic spas pierced through: Brooklyn meets guy, Jenny gets jealous before Jenny meets guy, kissing happens, and hearts are broken... *At least not my heart.*

I made my way towards Sean, a very buff, very tan Scottish man who had clearly been tipped off about my arrival.

"You must be Jenny." He nodded.

"Ah, so you've heard of me? I mean I guess I'm a big deal, but I didn't think people knew me in Thailand." I took a seat next to Sean, who found my comment amusing.

Sean was a marine biologist obtaining his scuba diving license so he could study sea life around the United Kingdom. He picked up MMA fighting while in Thailand, and after hours of chatting and dancing, he also picked me up on his yellow motorcycle for a ride back to his house.

"Hop onto my Lamborghini." He smiled as he handed me a helmet for his Yamaha.

When he led us to his bedroom, he offered me water and began playing a familiar tune of psychedelic rock.

"You like Tame Impala?" Sean asked.

I smiled and nodded, continuing to nod my head to the beat of my new favorite artist. Sean the scuba diver then laid me down and began his descent.

In the morning, Sean took me back to my resort before his job, where I found Brooklyn laying on a couch in the lobby.

"Brooklyn!" I gasped. Her head slowly lifted from the throw pillow.

"Jenny..." She said as she fluttered her eyes open.

"Bastien took me back in the middle of the night because he had an early morning dive, and you had our key, so I was locked out."

"O shit, I'm so sorry!" I said in all sincerity.

"It's ok, I shouldn't have gone home with him. He was cute and all, but so narcissistic. I mean... no oral!" Brooklyn rolled up into a seat. "Woo. I'm cold. Let's go to the room. I need a real nap." Brooklyn said, half asleep.

After a few more hours of rest, Brooklyn and I spent the day hiking up a dormant volcano; a verdant mountain laced in palm trees and waterfalls. We picked up mangosteen at a produce market, which have a hard, plum-like exterior and sweet bulbs of juicy flesh inside. To end the day, we paid 600 baht (nearly 20 USD) for an hour-long massage on the beach as the sun set. We were in bliss.

Disease and evil had no place here. Koh Chang's crystal blue waters diluted my bulimic brain, erasing my recent health scare. Wanderlust suppressed my demonic desires like a magic wand. *Poof* I was cured.

During that weekend in Thailand, I loved what I was seeing, and I loved who I was with. I was relieved to take a trip to the ocean opposed to the emergency room. I was lucky to visit Thailand with a trusted friend who could navigate us around the country, and lucky to have the means to afford the flight. I was lucky to be able to hike up waterfalls and hop on the back of a Yamaha. But most of all, I was lucky to be alive.

...

With a few months left in my teaching contract, money was tighter than my largest pair of leggings. I was spending every won on travel, food, and soju. My first weekend back from Thailand, I went out drinking with Selena and her friends at a swanky bar in Itaewon. Lime green moss coated the walls, where roped swings hung from the ceilings. We drank frozen, fruity cocktails with umbrella garnishes and trailed off to a jazz bar covered in records. To end, we stumbled inside a chimaek restaurant for one last beer and a basket of fried chicken.

"Shit!" I mumbled into my wing.

"What?" Selena asked.

"I'm *the worst* vegan." I pouted.

Selena and the group laughed and patted my back.

"It's ok if you're not vegan, Jenny." Selena assured me.

That was the end of my vegan streak. I went straight back to dairy, consuming and expelling at excelling rates. My bank account suffered in keeping up with my hunger, so I looked for alternative ways to fund my frenzies. I started to auction off everything in my apartment, which wasn't much. After stripping myself from material possessions, I offered up the last resources I had: my brain and my body.

Initially, I posted an ad as an English tutor, fully aware that doing so was a violation of my contract, but the risk of prosecution was low. This spark of mischief got me wondering at what lengths I would go to exploit myself. I had already kissed death. So why not try my hand as an escort? With five million men living in Seoul, I figured a few of them might be interested in an American companion. If I had hit rock bottom with my hives, then there was no place lower to go. My self-loathing led to disrespect and disconnection. I was so desperate to add value to my body, that I was willing to let someone else pay for it.

After clicking through online forums, I found a site that matched Korean men with foreign escorts. Writing my ad felt no different than setting up a dating profile, as my intent had always been indifferent. I wanted men to find me desirable, yet I never expected a response. I could cast the bait, but I didn't know how to reel in the catch.

Because God works in mysterious and comical ways, an offer for both tutoring and prostitution appeared within minutes of each other. This forced me to snap out of my internal crisis, shut down my promiscuous promotion, and reply to Mrs. Emma Park.

...

Emma Park and I agreed to meet on a Sunday afternoon for an initial session with her twin preteen daughters, Stella and Sasha. When she spotted me in her white BMW, she parked in the middle of traffic and stepped out in a fur coat which weighed more than she did.

"Nice to meet you" Emma said in a slow, practiced pace.

She drove me to her apartment building, which could not have been more than five years old. She led me through a hallway with marble floors and minimalist decor. One floor up, Emma opened the doors to her impeccably clean, modern apartment filled with silver furnishings and white accents. Down the hall, the twins waited for us by a charcuterie plate in the kitchen. The girls were timid, respectful, and kind with their bright, brown eyes.

"Tea?" Emma offered, pointing to her pink porcelain set.

Although technically considered 'the help,' I felt pampered. The Park women seemed at ease and the gig was a breeze. Plus, I got snacks. *I could get used to this.*

After three tutoring sessions, Emma asked if I'd be interested in teaching her friend Lisa Lee, a mother of toddlers who lived on the floor above the Park family.

Lisa was just as lovely as Emma, and immediately welcomed me as one of her own. Tutoring soon became much more than a paycheck, it was time in my week where I felt belonging. Also, snacks. I loved the snacks. I'd grown tired of nursery rhymes at the hagwon, so it was refreshing to lead lessons on current events. I found a database with short articles, choosing topics covering fast fashion, the wealth gap crises and mental health. With these reading assignments, I could connect to my pupils on a deeper level.

By Christmas, The Parks and the Lees invited me over to feast on unconventional holiday foods and open gifts I had no expectation of receiving. The husbands drank Cass Korean beer and poured chilled soju out of a glass decanter, which was a pleasant change from the plastic bottles I regularly chugged on the streets. We ate gummy rice cakes, sugared potato chips, and gourmet pizza drizzled in shrimp and French fries.

None of these traditions made sense to me, summing up an adequate conclusion for a dysfunctional year. Take away all the customs and cultural differences, all the K-Pop and ginseng tea. Strip me of the pride I gained from living abroad only to learn one vital thing: wherever I go, there I am. And sometimes, we don't get what we want, rather, we are surrounded by the people we need.

One frigid night in Seoul, Selena and I sipped on cheap lager in a vacant bar, enabling space for me to admit something I had held back since that first day we met in Seoraksan.

"I can't believe my contract is ending." I said.

"Any chance you'll renew?" Selena asked.

"No, I can't." I said.

"You can't? Did something happen at your hagwon?"

"No, like, *I* can't. I hardly made it through this year." I said.

"Was the school that bad?" Selena asked.

"The school was fine. But I'm not." I said.

Selena tipped her head, "what do you mean?"

"I'm, um... I'm bulimic. And it got really bad this year." I said.

"Oh, Jen." Selena reached out for my hand.

"I'm doing... better. But I've been severely depressed. And I'm telling you this because you've been a really good friend to me, truly. I didn't think I deserved your friendship, so thank you. Thank you for your kindness."

"What? Jen! Of course! I had no idea this was going on... you always seem so happy and so confident." Selena consoled me.

"I uh... am really good at seeming a certain way."

Selena and I finished our beers and walked back to the subway where she squeezed onto my puffer coat before my train arrived. I felt a bit lighter when I returned to my subway stop. Despite having the plan and cash in hand, I cooked dinner at my apartment and went to sleep.

...

With three weeks left in the school year, I asked Sunny about the details of my pension plan. According to my contract, I would receive the second half of my airfare to Korea, a full month's severance pay, and my housing deposit worth 600 USD. Overall, I anticipated $2,700 in my checking account once I left the country, along with my last month's pay. But when I sat down with Sunny to inquire about my leave, she froze behind her desk.

"Also, Sunny, when is my replacement teacher arriving?" I asked as Sunny frantically typed on her phone.

"If the new English teacher arrives early, I'd be happy to offer her my apartment as I can stay with a neighbor before my flight." I ventured, trying to catch her eye.

Sunny ignored me, then lifted the phone to her ear and shooed me out with her free hand. The next morning at work, Sunny waited for me by my desk. This was odd, considering her usual work hours started sometime after lunch.

"Okay, Jenny, we go upstairs." She led me to her office and shut the door. My chest burned, but I hadn't purged in days. The office suddenly seemed so big and vacant. The lights shone bright on her bulky desk and laptop. Sunny looked older than I remembered. It dawned on me that I hadn't sat down with her since my first week nearly a year ago. Beyond that, we rarely spoke. No evaluations, nothing. All my feedback from my Korean colleagues was pleasant and positive. Given the approval from teachers who observed my classes, I assumed there was no need for the principal to intervene. After all, Sunny seemed not to care.

"Jenny. There is no pension plan." She barked.

My stomach started churning, and it wasn't from overeating.

"What do you mean? It's in my contract." I responded.

"No! No contract!" She yelled. Her thick black bangs started rattling around her flushed skin.

"You steal from me!" She yelled louder.

I knew exactly what she meant and wanted to explain.

"I see you on CCTV! Jenny Teacher, then no Jenny Teacher!"

Sunny was right, I hadn't been going to the Play Cafe for the past month, as I was fed up with toddlers crying at my foreign face and their parents insisting that I leave them alone.

"Sunny, I'm sorry about the Play Cafe. But it was not a part of my contract."

"NO! No contract! You are done. No pay for February. No pension. You leave now."

I nearly vomited there on her desk, as it was mid-February and I had plans to travel until April. Those few thousand dollars of pension were my sole asset for supporting myself as I made my way home to America.

"But what about my classes? What about my students?" I asked as I held back tears.

"No English today. You are done."

I picked up my backpack and tried talking to my Korean colleagues as Sunny escorted me out of her building. But the other teachers avoided my plea and stared at Sunny fearfully, as they all knew something I didn't.

On my walk home I released an ugly, loud cry before plotting to get my dignity and my pension back. It dawned on me that both Tess and the teacher before her hadn't completed a full year at the hagwon, each breaching their contract, which expelled them from a pension. Sunny never had to pay them their exit rates. And here I was, inquiring about mine. I may have been disloyal for leaving the Play Cafe but dammit, I gave my best to my students. Sunny could hold the CCTV tapes against me, but I wasn't about to leave without a fight.

I called Ava, who knew someone with a similar experience. They turned me to a Facebook group of lawyers sharing rights and resources for teachers, as hagwon owners were notorious for taking advantage of their foreign employees and often manipulated their teaching contracts during the last month of the agreement.

"Turn around and go back to work," Ava warned me. "Sunny is looking for a viable reason to fire you, so she's telling you to leave for proof that you're not at work. Just go back and sit at your desk. If she doesn't let you teach, that gives you more time to fight for your case."

I walked back to the hagwon and unlocked the door with the keypad, signaling the alarm.

Bora ran down to warn me. "Jenny Teacher... Sunny said no-"

I cut my colleague off and smiled, "Sunny said a lot of things. She said to not teach so I will sit here, ok?" I pointed to my desk and settled down. My colleague walked away to avoid conflict with her boss who was now storming down the stairs.

"Jenny! What are you doing?" Sunny fumed.

"I am sitting at work, and I will do so until February 28, as written in my contract." I said boldly. The stare-off began, and I held my ground. As my dad might say, *he didn't raise no wimp.*

It worked. Sunny's fair skin blushed red before she stomped back to her office. Over the next few hours, I contacted Korean lawyers and researched my conditions. Multiple law professionals recommended that I take my contract to the Department of Labor, where I could file my case and threaten to sue Sunny if she breached my teaching agreement. During this time, I wrote a letter to Sunny explaining my homesickness, my depression, and my apology for missing Play Cafe hours. I included a note about how hurt I was by her expulsion at work. Then I sent the letter to one of Ava's Korean coworkers, who agreed to translate it for me out of sympathy.

That night I scrubbed my apartment dry. I had an inkling Sunny would find any speck of dirt and try to hold it against my security deposit. I spent hours on my knees, using a sponge to soak up all the impurities I had discharged over the course of the year.

I woke up early that next morning, ready to face the wrath of Sunny's response over my threat to sue. On my train ride to the Department of Labor, thoughts of my plan potentially backfiring rushed through my head. I envisioned myself broke and stranded in Korea.

What if Sunny fights back? What if she convinces the authorities that I had done something illegal? Had I done anything illegal? Could they arrest me for skipping out on a few Play Cafe shifts? Would I be thrown in jail and left to rot in Asia?

My breath shortened as I drew out this illusion, depleting much oxygen to my brain. Months had passed since my last dose of Klonopin, as my prescriptions put me in a dream-state which inevitably turned into a binging nightmare. Defenseless on the train, I felt a panic attack coming, puffing into my scarf to muffle my cries. Luckily, before my anxiety sent me into full terror, I snapped back when the train stopped. As I checked the map for navigation, interpreting the web of rainbow lines forced me to focus on my destination and step out of the dark destiny I had fabricated in my mind.

A glass wall separated myself from the clerk at the Department of Labor, where I watched sweat form on my forehead in the vague reflection. With all my paperwork presented, the clerk called Sunny from their desk.

"Please God, *please*, if you exist, allow Sunny to show some mercy for me today." I repeated in my head.

I stared at the clerk in despair, unable to translate anything until she hung up the phone.

"Yes. Ms. Martin. Your employer has agreed to pay your pension in full. Please keep my card if anything changes. I cannot, however, determine the result of your security deposit as that will be dependent on the property owner of your apartment."

I sighed in relief and thanked the clerk graciously. I had won the war, with one last battle to fight.

When it came time for my housing inspection, I brought along my neighbor Mena, a Korean mother I had befriended while sipping soju one summer night outside a 7-11.

Mena defended me as Sunny and the landlord dubbed my apartment "too dirty" for them to refund my security deposit. Mena and Sunny really went at each other, yelling in Korean over whether the mold in my closet was my doing. Watching them, I cursed myself for not taking 'before' photos the day I moved in. Eventually, I stepped into their brawl and told them it didn't matter anymore, that Sunny could keep her security deposit and the satisfaction of taking advantage of a foreigner.

Taking advantage of a foreigner. I emphasized that line in my translated letter to Sunny, studying her reaction as I made her read the letter in front of me during my last day of school. I wrote about leaving my family to work for her and asked that she put herself in my shoes. I challenged her to take our turbulent parting into consideration when laying down expectations for the next English teacher. I spoke for myself and the other English teachers as curious, young expatriates looking to immerse ourselves in Korean culture. Leaving *everything* behind for a chance to create a new life in a different part of the world. The experience we have at our hagwon is one of the greatest impressions we'll have of Korea, which we will carry back to our home country. And that impression is a major reflection of the principal.

I could tell that Ava's friend did an excellent job of translating my emotive message, as Sunny's face tightened with each sentence she scanned across the page.

"Ok. Thank you." Sunny nodded sternly and pointed to the door.

"Thank you." I reciprocated and reached out my hand. Sunny complied, and I gripped her hand tight.

...

In the last weeks of my contract, Sunny continued to exclude me from class, so I spent my free time creating YouTube travel videos at my desk. While Sunny tried to subvert my departure away from the students, I refused to leave without hugging every kid goodbye. On my last day, I gifted each child with a card.

A student named David gripped my leg tight as his English-speaking mom retrieved her son from school.

"Jenny! You are still here! David has been talking about you all week, saying that you had left." Said the mom.

"Awe, that's so sweet. Actually, today is my last day." I smiled back.

"Best of luck to you. This has been hard on David. He adored you. Last week he came home crying because you were leaving, and I had to explain that you were going home to be with your family. Then, a plane went by, and David pointed up to the sky and asked me, 'Is that Jenny Teacher?' It was the cutest thing."

I glanced down at David, now nestled between his mom and his retired English teacher. I saved my tears for my walk home when I thought, maybe I had made an impact after all.

...

When I look at my pictures from Korea, I scroll through a sea of green mountain trails and coastal waters. I see myself smiling under a pagoda or laughing behind a bottle of soju. My photos represent a life of adventure, framing the main subject to appear as a courageous, confident one.

As people would ask me about my year in Asia, I'd respond, "Great! Let me show you a clip of my kiddos." But the more I processed my pain, the more my reaction started to shift with my awareness. It took twelve months to admit to people that 'Korea was the craziest, hardest year of my life... It was the year I didn't die." And while I may tailor this response to whoever is listening, I try to be brutally honest. There's no need to sugar coat a season where everything I ate was sugar coated. I left home for a city strange to me, landing in my own unique hell. I bought a timeshare to rock bottom, invested in my disease. The entire time I thought no one was watching, that no one cared. And in this isolation, I started to see there was something greater than me looking out for my protection.

At the eye of the storm, I meditated for the first time. I journaled on topics other than what I ate, including foul thoughts not suitable for young eyes to read. I prayed. Not entirely sure to whom, but I prayed because that seemed like a better option than giving up entirely.

I traveled over an ocean to prove to my friends, my family, and my followers that I could escape my problems, only to learn that my problems swell as I travel, just like my feet during a 14-hour flight.

I left Seoul bitter and physically bigger. While I stopped weighing myself after the scale reached 88 kilograms, I would guess that I passed 200 pounds by the time I departed. Between my final "annyeong" to my students and my flight out of Korea, I spent a week living off chocolate bars, ramen, and cigarettes. During this stint, I slept on the floor of my neighbor's, Alana. I drank Cass beer and blew cigarette smoke out of Alana's window, slowly packing my life back into the two suitcases I carried into Seoul. I flicked the ask of the last cigarette into a plastic cup.

"I think I'll take up smoking to suppress my appetite." I joked.

Alana looked down at me with pity, sighing out her parting words:

"Take care of yourself, Jenny."

Homecoming

After my third attempt to withdraw Vietnamese Dong from the airport ATM, I managed to move around enough money to pay for my entrance visa at Noi Bai International. Thank God for my pension and credit line. My homecoming had begun. A weight lifted off my dampened spirit in Hanoi as I said "good riddance" to Seoul and disposed of my winter coat into the trash. No need for a down jacket in the jungle. During my cab ride into town, I watched braids of telephone wire thicken between the jumbled buildings, indicating proximity to the Old Quarter where my friend Erica was waiting for me at our hotel.

Erica had played volleyball in college, where we met and took up partying as a serious sport. She was now working in Boston and had drained every hour of her PTO on this trip to Vietnam and Thailand. Tall and beautiful, Erica looked fitter than ever when I spotted her from the hotel entrance. While she subscribed to the 'work hard, play hard' mentality with me in school, Erica matured out of late nights and darties. (Day Parties). She had a respectable job, a serious boyfriend, and an adult volleyball league that she traveled with on the weekends. All I had was a suitcase of clothes I could hardly fit into, and *just enough* money to click my ruby slippers back to Kansas. After my fifth beer on a Ha Long Bay overnight cruise, I turned to Erica as we watched the sunset:

"I'm sorry you have to see me like this. It's not fair for you to fly all this way to stand next to your fat friend." I caved.

We leaned over the ship's railing, peering over the infamous rock formations that filled up the bay. Across the horizon, dozens of limestone karsts sat erect out of the lagoon, draped in vegetation, clouded by a light layer of fog. This was the Instagram moment I had imagined, standing thirty pounds lighter, in a bikini next to my fit best friend. Instead, clouds muddled the sky and light rain kept us covered up under pink ponchos.

"Jenny! Don't ever say such a thing! I am so happy to be here, and I'm so happy to see you. I have always thought of you as beautiful, and I still do. Because you *are beautiful, ok?*"

She seemed annoyed at first, before her face softened.

"Hey..." Erica lifted her poncho to reveal her long, lean limbs and torso. "Let's get in." She nodded at the water. I blushed at the thought of taking off my clothes. At either corner of the upper deck, 18-year-old British boys congregated with their drinks as they celebrated spring break. "Jenny... Don't worry about those guys. You'll never see them again." Erica assured me.

Like a switch, my "fuck-it" mentality kicked in. But this time, my lack of fucks boosted my self-assurance.

"You're right. Let's go!"

Erica helped to lift me to the edge of the railing and kept grip of my right hand.

"One...Two...Three!"

We flung off the edge, like spider monkeys jumping from tree to tree. The crisp water removed the remorse I had built around my body. Much like how I spent every childhood summer, Erica and I repeatedly circled up the ship's ladder to spring off the ledge. We laughed like kids, drawing the British boys to join in. For a moment, I forgot about the size of my belly and just let myself *be.*

After cruising around the emerald isles of Ha Long Bay, Erica and I hopped on a flight to Bangkok to meet no other than my ultimate travel buddy, Brooklyn. That night, Erica, Brooklyn, Brooklyn's sister, and I partied along the backpacker's strip of Khaosan Road, dancing in crowded streets while waving rum buckets in the air. Around 2am, we found a string of massage chairs lined up for patrons to opt for a late-night foot rub. It was glorious. From the buzzing streets of Bangkok, we cabbed straight to the airport for our 5am flight to Koh Samui. There, we would spend two days relaxing beside pristine beaches before a hedonic night at the infamous Full Moon Party.

Back in the 1980's, a group of tourists set up a party on a remote island in Thailand, dancing into the sunrise with plenty of booze and a boombox or two. Whatever these backpackers were up to, they must have fancied themselves. Because the same group returned the same time the following year, bringing more friends. The tradition continued into the 90's and has now evolved into a monthly event sanctioned on the beach of Koh Phangan, all to license alcohol sales, centralize noise pollution, and profit off of illicit drug use.

"Drugs! Brooklyn! Where can we buy some drugs?" I asked as I sipped a mimosa at lunch, counting down the minutes before it was socially acceptable to drink anything harder.

"Easy… Jenny. Drugs won't be a problem here. Just chill for now. We can start scouting at sunset." Alarmed, Brooklyn could tell I wasn't just itching for a high, but to soar far, far away.

Soon, the sun would set, inviting the beauties and the beasts to come out to play. My girlfriends and I set up a spot on the beach to begin the metamorphosis. With every mimosa, I felt less plump sitting next to my toned friends. I took neon paint to Erica's lean arms, dabbing tribal patterns up and down her limbs. She reciprocated, and when the electric designs had dried, I had successfully camouflaged.

I added floral details to Erica's face when a group of men walked up to our blanket. A little drunk and heavily concentrating on the body art, I missed most of the conversation Brooklyn had initiated with these men. Eventually, I put my brush down and looked up at our visitors, dressed in crisp, linen button ups, bright swim trunks and designer sunglasses. Late thirties, tanned skin, dark hair. They were visiting from Pakistan, all owning multiple businesses. A handsome man kneeled beside me and asked for some paint for an exchange of a sip from his rum bucket.

"Knock yourself out." I offered him my brush and he held out a straw.

"Same to you. This is MDMA."

Oh, hell yea!

MDMA. What. A. Drug. The only other time I had rolled molly was at nineteen during a Dayglow Party, which, similarly subjected participants to copious amounts of neon paint.

Remembering that slimy, spectacular night from my sophomore year, I leaned in for a gulp from this stranger's bucket.

"Isn't MDMA like, highly illegal in Thailand? How did you get it through border control?" I asked.

The man placed a small plastic bag in my hand.

"You can pay for *anything* in Thailand," chuckled the man.

"Thanks for the paint!" The group of men tipped their heads and walked out to the shore, taking their buckets of drugs and leaving a baggie behind. *Hello, Molly. We meet again.*

"Jenny. Listen to me. Be *very* careful with this." Warned Brooklyn as she passed the bag into my hands while we switched places in a dingy bathroom stall. My friends made it clear they were concerned about my mental health, probably because I had complained all trip about my body and mental health.

I locked the door and looked closely at the crystals, which resembled black sand. *I'm pretty sure that's not what my molly looked like last time. But what the hell, what could possibly go wrong?*

I licked my finger and stuck it into the granular substance, scooping up broken shards and scrubbed them into my gums. I gagged. *Tastes like battery acid.*

There was a considerable chunk left in the bag, along with loose residue. I took that little black rock and swallowed it whole, tucked the bag into my swimsuit top and rushed out of the stall. Brooklyn stopped to confiscate the remaining drugs, trading it for a rum bucket to wash down the bitter taste from my gums.

"Give it here, Jenny" Brooklyn held out her hand, and I reached for the bag in my boob. We both knew better than to let me hold onto the drugs, though no one at the time could have predicted what would happen next.

The sky dimmed from pink to black as tiki torches lit up along the beach, initiating a howling spirit for the Full Moon Party. Kiosks lined up by the sand selling rum buckets and glo sticks. Hundreds of young people huddled in front of DJ booths and fire blowers. A tanned, ripped young man parted a sea of dancers with his torch, hypnotizing his audience to the stream of EDM blasting in the background.

Mesmerized, I could hear my friends beside me, but all I could see were surges of light. Voices began to warp and soon all I could see was the beat of the music. A double take of neon beams swayed towards me, interrupting my vision. So, I kept my eyes closed as we danced, only opening them to check in with my friends.

"Woah! Where did you get it?" Neon strangers asked as I followed Erica out of the crowd, tightly gripping onto her shoulder. Too high to respond, I just kept smiling up at the sky, bumping my head to the techno beats. *Wherever I got it, there was none left to share.*

"Jenny! Look at me!" As soon as we exited a tight crowd, Erica turned around, startled. She investigated my pupils, making sure I still had white left in my eyes. I took a deep breath and looked up at my friend. Two images of Erica glanced down at me in despair. Wait a minute. I wasn't just cross faded. I was cross eyed.

Damnit.

I shut my eyes and smiled to my friends, "I'll be fine" I promised as I continued dancing.

"No, Jen! You're not fine. Look at me." asked Erica.

With my feet dug firmly into the sand, I started tapping at my temples like one would bang an old television to fix a broken screen. Keeping my eyes shut, I took one long inhale, releasing sweet, sweet neurotransmitters to my brain. And when I opened my eyes, a fork full of Pad Thai was being shoved into my mouth.

"Holy hell! She's alive!" exclaimed Brooklyn.

"Guys… are we?" I could see for the first time in what felt like hours. The four of us huddled around a picnic table on the outskirts of the party. Then, something in my mouth began to sting.

"We are still at the party, Jen. Just sobering you up before we head back out." Brooklyn assured me.

"What's with the lemons?" I licked the sour from my lips and pointed down at the pile of yellow wedges.

"Someone suggested we give you citrus to kill your high, so we sat you down and had you finish a whole plate." Erica chimed in. She broke a smile, then again put on her "serious" face.

"O shit, guys. I am so, so sorry you had to babysit me. I totally ruined the night." I looked at our table, covered in lemon peels and a half-eaten plate of Pad Thai.

My friends sighed to agree that yes, I depended on their care and yes, I burdened the night.

"We thought we lost you. You can't take drugs from strange men, even if they're millionaires." Said Brooklyn.

"You took them, too!" I argued.

"Yea, but we didn't go cross-eyed."

Everyone laughed.

"Seriously, Jenny, you're too pretty to have your eyes get stuck like that forever." Brooklyn smiled as she led the four of us back into the crowd, where we danced soberly for the rest of the night.

"Yo! What happened to my body paint? Did I jump in the water?" I looked down at my naked limbs. My friends shot me a look that said, "No, dumbass," and I excused myself to grab some much needed water.

After sweating off the spoiled molly, I endured a different type of woozy: jet lag. I spent a day in the sky, soaring west towards Europe to crash in Madrid before a week in London, staying with friends who were gracious in providing necessities: shelter and booze. This helped to stretch out the two thousand dollars I had left to my name, as I was financing much of this trip on my credit card. I figured my homecoming would be one last hurrah before facing the "real world," where I'd find a "big girl job," or at least something to help pay off my growing debt and allow for more travel.

My connecting flight to America issued a long layover in Reykjavik, where I was too broke to do anything besides tiptoe around the coastal town and scout for a meal that wouldn't cost more than the flight through Iceland itself. Arriving in the late afternoon, the Nordic town of pale buildings with red rooftops started to cool down, as if looking through a blue, somber filter. Walking to the edge of the port city, I studied the black waters, wondering when I'd be able to experience Iceland the "right" way, with excursions to waterfalls and the Instagramable Blue Lagoon. On this trip, "my way" looked like a 16-bedroom dorm in a hostel which charged extra for a blanket and pillow upon arrival. With the little change I had allotted for dinner, my cheapest option was a burger and fries from a bodega.

I'll start being vegan again when I'm home with a job.

With that goal in mind, I bought a few chocolate bars and walked back to the hostel.

I'll start being healthy again when I'm home with a job.

The next morning, I boarded a flight to Chicago, sitting between a plus-size model who had just finished a gig in Ireland and a woman who had met up with her online boyfriend for the first time in Barcelona. The model bought our row a glass of wine and offered to drive me from the airport to my friend's house. Refreshed, I reveled in my luck.

This is it, Jen. This is your homecoming. Free wine, free rides, and free advice from a gorgeous woman heavier than you who is getting paid *to do something she loves. Now it's your turn to make something of yourself.*

In Chicago, I stayed with my college friend Liam, who is both very smart, very sarcastic, and very, very, gay. Liam had a full agenda for us. I passed on watching the premiere of "RuPaul's Drag Race," but I did get out to watch our alma mater play in the NCAA national basketball championship during a little tournament Americans call 'March Madness.' My disinterest in sports had crashed steadily since my final swim meet of junior year, but basketball is one game I can follow through overtime. Throw some ice-cold drafts into the mix, and you've got yourself a true fan.

That is… unless… could it be??

I sat front and center at the dubbed alumni bar in Chicago. And sure, I had surrounded my barstool with several alumni, but one face never made its way towards my seat. For those few painful hours watching the game, I could see his reflection in the bar's mirrored backsplash where he stood with his now fiancé. Keeping my eyes fixed to the screen, I made damn sure Chad wouldn't see me in my current state. My weight gain was too much of a burden for my self-esteem.

I was drunk by the time the game started, and I needed to be hammered when it ended. Not because our team was losing, but because I was humiliated to be seen in the body I had marred over three years of neglect.

When Chad met me, I was skin and bones. But after years of binging, I saw myself as a blob hiding under a sweatshirt. I left America in peace knowing that no one would know who I was, where I came from, or what I used to look like. But there at that alumni bar, I was high fiving a room full of people from my past. While I recognized their faces, I knew they were looking at a much different woman.

That Jenny Martin… she was hot in college, but damn, did she let herself go.

This line ran through my thoughts all game long, as I conspired more reasons to loathe my body. I didn't want to be seen looking like this, let alone caught by the eyes of an old lover. I ordered another beer at the bar and drank it up quickly, avoiding Chad at all costs.

Maybe if I forget this night, so will they.

After the game, Liam wanted to stay out in Boystown, so I walked back to his apartment alone. The midnight air offered tranquility, knowing I would soon be safe with Netflix, hiding away from humanity.

That Jenny Martin… Is what I'm sure 'they' were all saying.

Damn, did she let herself go.

After a week in Chicago, I packed for the last big stretch of my global tour. There was no room to feel sorry for myself as I was flying into a corner of the world where anything was possible, and everyone is a star. And that's the City of Angels. The city of *Los Angeles.*

Initially, I planned to stay in San Francisco with a friend for a week, but that friend moved to New York a month before my flight. I contemplated wandering around America's most expensive city on my own or renting a car to drive south and stay with a high school friend in Orange County. Seeing that I had friends, free accommodation, and fresh ground to explore in L.A., I opted for the hills over the bay. My flight from Chicago landed at 2am in San Francisco, where I picked up my first rental car and slid it south towards Carmel-by-the-Sea. Under the starlight, I parked along the beach and reclined the driver's seat to nap. When I woke up to the sunrise, I had scored a front row seat to the Pacific Ocean.

Look out Hollywood, I'm coming for ya.

Elated, I ran out to the untouched beach, where I was the first to make footprints in the sand. Boulders scattered along the coast, where the waves rolled in closer and closer to my feet. I felt an overwhelming urge to call my dad, of whom I hadn't talked to for a couple months after Trump got elected. I put our political opinions aside to show off to my father that I had made it to California, a state he condemns as a host for artsy-fartsy liberals.

"Look at this beach!" I shouted during our Facetime call.

"My... that's something else." He said, looking pleased, but not as enthused as I was. I cried out of contentment, enthralled by nature's beauty.

"Dad, I'm so inspired here. Mark my words, I *will* move to the West Coast one day."

"Well. Good for you, Jenny. That's fine if you want to move to California.... all you need is money."

I hung up the call without getting hung up on his advice. Not everyone living in Cali was a movie star or a millionaire; people made it work in any industry. And while I was still unsure of what kind of career I wanted, I would make it work, too.

I stretched out a four-hour drive down the Pacific Coast Highway into seven, stopping to hike and photograph the monstrous beauty of Big Sur. On the second night, I stayed in Santa Barbara to meet up with a woman who had gone to my college, graduated in my class, was friends with Liam and others from my circle, yet had only known me through my social media. Her name was Claire.

"Jenny! It's so nice to meet you!" Claire picked me up from my downtown hostel and took us to the main pier and a popular pizza parlor. Before we met up, I was nervous about catfishing this woman for our friend date, as she had only known me through highly edited photos. And photos, in which I did a damn good job of hiding my weight.

But as we talked, Claire looked at me with sincerity etched on her face, "I've loved following all your adventures since graduation. You've inspired me to teach English in Asia, too."

Claire and I spent the next four hours eating pizza and splitting a bottle of wine back at her apartment. What I originally expected to be a short engagement with someone who knew me off a profile page evolved into an evening of dream-casting, storytelling, and of course, a bit of college gossip.

"Wait, so you hung out with all those girls living off Clemons Street?" I asked Claire, speaking of a house full of chicks who were as pretty as they were petty.

"Yes! I can't believe we never met. But yo, I don't speak to any of them anymore. And from Instagram, it looks like they don't speak to one another, either." Said Claire.

"Dude... they've always been catty. Last time I spoke to Brittany, she asked me why I was still talking to Mara and told me that Mara only likes me because of my lifestyle." I spouted over my third glass of Santa Barbara red.

"Jenny, you do seem like you have quite the lifestyle, but like, that's not enough to keep a friendship." Claire responded.

Claire was right. I wasn't sure who were friends, and who were fans at this point. I wasn't even sure which lifestyle they were after because at this point, it was all a facade.

The next day, I was well rested, showered, and set to tackle the impending L.A. traffic on the 101. While I had a music to listen to, I played through the stereotypes about California fed to me while growing up in the Midwest:

Living on the coast is too expensive. Stay central or burden your grandkids to pay off your mortgage after you die.

Los Angeles is too crowded. You'll spend all your time in traffic and all your money on rent.

Everyone in L.A. is fake. They're all hungry for money and fame.

These are direct quotes from my friends, my parents, and my parents' friends, who warned me to be cautious of greedy liberals and vain entertainers. And while movies were a central part of my childhood, I strongly disassociated actors from real people, as anyone famous was surely from a different planet. After all, I grew up during the golden era of paparazzi, when all my Disney stars started getting DUI's. In high school, I would set the dinner table while watching Access Hollywood, where Mario Lopez treated every celebrity like the Queen. My humble mother would finish seasoning her chicken etouffee, hinting at the successful recipe, reminding me that "men like a woman who can cook."

...

"Hey Jen. Park in the lot near the coffee shop and I'll ring you up. My friend Olivia just arrived for the weekend, too. You'll love her." Luke, my guy friend from high school, buzzed me up to the top level of his building just a mile away from the beach. Luke had been living in L.A. for three years now, working night shifts in cargo operations and making one hell of a living.

My tanned, Asian-Pacific friend opened the door, still fit with a head of curly hair I once used to swoon over with my raging teenage hormones. I hugged Luke, relieved to see someone who felt like home. I rolled my luggage through Luke's chic apartment and saw an elegant, long-legged blonde sitting on the couch.

"Welcome to Cali, sweetie!" Olivia jumped up to hug me, and I tried to stay cool around this gorgeous creature.

Between unpacking my things, I made small talk with Olivia and asked her what I should wear for our upcoming night out.

"This is L.A., honey. No one cares what you wear." Olivia laughed in all seriousness.

Keeping that in mind, I picked out my favorite funky sweatshirt and a pair of leggings, both of which hid my tummy quite well. I joined Luke and

Olivia and their chiseled actor friend to a club in Orange County, where the candy-colored disco floor ate away all my tummy woes. Around 3am, I followed Luke back to his couch where we spoke of high aspirations as we came down from partying.

"What's next for the world traveler?" Luke asked. I paused, expecting this question a dozen times over during my return to Kansas City. I was tired of filtering my life of who I thought others wanted me to be. Luckily, with Luke, I could just be... *me*.

"Well... if you haven't noticed, I've gained a lot of weight. Like, a lot a lot. I have an eating disorder, no doubt." The vodka tonics really lubricated my response. Never had I told a *boy* this before, and it felt liberating.

"What I really need to do when I get home is heal. Get some help, you know? Work on my mental health." I concluded.

"Jenny, don't stress about your weight. We've all gained weight since high school. You look great." Luke said in a sweet yet obligatory tone. He wanted to comfort me, though I wasn't fishing for compliments.

"Yeah, but it's more than what I look like. I need to ground down and get to the root of why I'm so obsessed with eating. And why I can't see how others see me. You know?" I started staring up to the ceiling, ready to *go there*.

"Jenny, this is America. Everyone is obsessed with their bodies and food. You're not the only one."

"Exactly." The words emerged up my throat as I admitted something aloud for the first time. "Before I started restricting food, I wanted to be a counselor and help people with eating disorders, but that was before I got a *really bad* eating disorder. By college, I knew I'd write a book, and now I know what that book is going to be about."

"Oh yea?" Luke asked.

"Yea. It'll be my memoir. About traveling with an eating disorder. About trying to escape my problems, and how I've hid behind the camera instead of facing my disease. Like you said, our culture is *obsessed* with looks and yet, we're the fattest, sickest country in the world. I'm not the only person struggling. And I hope that by sharing my story I will help people to see that they are not alone." I finished my ramblings and gaped out to the corner of Luke's living room.

Luke tilted his head in the same direction, staring off into the dreamscape. "Do it. And when you get your book deal, be sure to have a guest room ready for me in your L.A. penthouse when we go out and celebrate."

The next morning Luke headed to a country music festival, which ain't my kinda music and surely wasn't how I wanted to spend my time in California. Instead, I followed Olivia and her friends to various hot spots in Los Angeles. This day drinking led me to question how my pretty, plastic peers perceived me. Though these peers were my ticket into Hollywood's nightclubs with free table service and primo MDMA, the kind that didn't make my eyes cross. But regardless of how clean the drugs were, the women intimidated me. I found myself at a pregame party with a group of girls who were half my dress size, all getting ready and trading clothes. As they tossed skimpy tops back and forth between bedrooms, I checked my makeup in the bathroom, disturbed by the girl I had to confront in the mirror.

Damnit, Jenny. If you could have just stuck to your diet and gym plan in Korea, you would look just like them. You don't deserve to be seen with these women.

"Oo, I love that lip color. You've got such a beautiful smile." A girl said as she grabbed her makeup bag off the vanity.

The flattery startled me. This woman was a stunt double by trade, and an athlete by default of this trade. I smiled back as I scanned her exceptionally toned body.

With that compliment, I shook off my weight woes. After hours of liquor, molly, and club bangers to dance to in our VIP booth, I shed my stereotypes about LA folk. I was worried that people would care about what I looked like, but they were busy caring about themselves. I drove seven hours into the City of Angels wondering how people would judge me, and it turned out I was the only one doing so.

I crashed at the stunt-double's house that night, then on a couch of a college acquaintance the next. Thanks to the internet, I met up with old friends willing to drive through traffic to catch up and talk travel. These friends came from all chapters of life and assured me that I wasn't as lonely or crazy as I felt. They listened compassionately when I told them the truth about my mental health and thanked me for my vulnerability. Despite how I was still overeating, this space for honesty lifted so much off my plate.

Of all the cities before, none had infused such a bolt of inspiration to light my path ahead. For it was here, in Los Angeles, I told people I wanted to write as a career. And here, for the first time, people validated this dream.

"Yes mami!"

"Go for it!"

"Yes, Jen! I love reading your blog. You are a great writer."

"My boss just published a book; do you want her email?"

In the Midwest, I was either too ashamed to admit my creative pursuits or shunned by my aspirations. A typical response from my parents on becoming an actor, writer or director was a pitiful stare and the reminder to "be realistic." But not here, not in L.A. When I told people about my dreams, they did not question me. They supported me. My mind was set. I'd head home to the Midwest and save up to move to La La Land. What could *possibly* get in the way of my plan this time?

While I waited at my gate at LAX, I put up a Facebook post asking if anyone knew of any restaurants hiring. I was hours away from my Kansas City homecoming, and I already sought a plan to get out. Los Angeles taught me that I could be an artist, so I would do as the artists do. I would wait tables, live with my parents, and save money so I could move to the big city and make it as a writer. No longer did I need to find myself by getting lost, as I finally knew what I was supposed to do: tell my story, *Jenny Eats the World.*

Emotionally Bankrupt

Within days of writing that Facebook post, I started serving at a bar and grill two miles from my parents' house. I had hoped my parents would be proud of me for securing work so quickly, but it turned out they were less than impressed to watch their college-educated daughter come home smelling like fries.

"It's just a buffer job while I find a *real* job." I lied. In truth, I was smoking weed out my bathroom window and making YouTube videos about my Asian adventures. It was during this phase of my creative renaissance that I listed prospective passion projects in my journal around the themes and titles of future vlogs and blog posts, spending hours into the night working on anything but my memoir. Editing content from Korea became so fun and fascinating as I spun parts of a tragic year into entertaining memories captured on film. Upon the 12 hours I'd spend on one 4-minute video, I started to appreciate every minute I lived in Asia, scene by scene.

I burned out after seven videos. And while I enjoyed the creative process, my parents questioned how the twenty views from grandma and friends would expand into a viable career. Even Liam, my corporate friend in Chicago who was photographing headshots on the side questioned the ROI for my time.

"You're very talented, Jenny. Your videos are good, but it's a saturated market for travel vloggers, and you're far away from monetizing anything on YouTube. But you're great with people... have you ever thought of HR?" Liam asked during a phone call.

Ugh. HR. Yes, I had taken an early morning HR class in college, often dozing off with post-practice fatigue. I didn't see a strong correlation (for myself, at least) between being a good people-person and being good in HR. I mean, you eventually let people down in that job, and after watching The Office, Toby Flenderson's character didn't exactly sell me on the position.

Besides, working HR in a corporate building felt too binding. I was a *creative,* thus required *creative freedom,* and kept on dreaming and drinking. Three years had passed since I called Kansas City "home," so upon arrival, I jumped straight into party mode with my friends from high school. This particular group of women had all graduated from the same college and were now on their second and third degrees. They were bright, responsible, and sophisticated in between tequila shots on the weekends. And while each of these women possess a beautiful, unique personality, I will refer to this group as a collective to protect personal information about the people who supported me during what came next.

However, there is one person from high school who stands apart from this collective. Bentley Foster and I grew up in the same neighborhood as kids, attached at the hip and drawn to each other's weirdness. She was all in for my nontraditional birthday parties, where I made my classmates summon spirits with a Ouija board and watch 90's horror films at twelve years old. Upon reflecting on our childhood, Bentley said that she loved me as a kid because I was the "only one crazier than she was."

But as we moved up to middle school, I focused on swimming and Bentley was more focused on boys, as the boys couldn't take their eyes off of her. She was popular, attending all the parties and participating in things most kids do when they're not swimming 25 hours a week. This distance continued throughout high school and our friendship ceased to exist when we left for college.

By our mid-20's, Bentley and I had not spoken in years, but we still followed one another on Instagram. She too had studied abroad in Europe, taught across America, and spent a season in Bali to complete her 200 Hour

Yoga Teacher Training. So, when she messaged me after I posted a blog titled, "Traveling to Escape Life," I was more than happy to rekindle a long-lost friendship. We were now both in Kansas City and made a date for drinks one afternoon.

"How the hell are you?!" Bentley reached her long limbs around me, looking effortlessly chic in her cream-colored top and black skinny jeans.

"I just have to say, I've never known someone to be *so real* online. I loved your post about mental health. It's refreshing to read something honest for once." Bentley flashed her pearly teeth with her sincere words.

In my post, "Traveling to Escape Life," I explained how I pulled a 'geographic' to hide from my problems and for the first time online, I wrote about my bulimia. Bentley then shared with me her past of crippling depression, the trauma she experienced while teaching in Miami, and her reformation from decreasing her drug use. After her stoner phase in college and the powders in Europe, Bentley sat in front of me clean, but not completely sober. Over a little wine, she became my newest guru.

As I spent time with Bentley, I also engaged with her big, beautiful family. Bentley's sister Reagan was just as cool and collected as I remembered her and was kicking major ass as a sales manager for a staffing agency. The more Reagan talked about the benefits and mobility of her company, the more that a desk job—or at least *this* desk job—seemed like a practical option over my stagnant life as a "starving" artist.

At the bar and grill, I was making next to nothing with $5 burgers and $2 tacos on my tickets. I left some weekend shifts with less than fifty dollars cash, so yea, a full-time job with benefits would make it far easier for me to balance my finances so I could focus on writing. I told myself I was too stressed over money for creativity to come through, so it only made sense for me to apply to a more stable situation.

When Regan referred me to her company, I noticed from LinkedIn that a dozen old classmates from high school were also working at the agency. My application took weeks to process, which left me wondering, *"If they could get a job here, why can't I?"*

When the interviews started, I left frustrated, questioning my competence like my interviewer had. On my fourth interview, I met with the COO, Izzy. Izzy met me in the reception lounge and led us into a room that barely fit two people, sitting me down with my resume in hand.

Izzy looked like she had just walked out of a J. Crew on the first day of spring, dressed head to toe in new arrivals. She forced a smile, and I smiled back, breathing steadily to hone in confidence and prepared for the best.

After the prerequisite small talk, Izzy jumped right in.

"Now I'll ask a series of questions that I ask everyone who walks through that door. Ready?"

I smiled in confirmation.

"What are your strengths?"

O geez, Izzy! Google declared that question antiquated!

It's ok, it's ok. I got a good one.

"My passion" I said with grace.

"I care. I care about doing a good job and I care about being the best. I've always been a hard worker and that laps back into wanting to be a top performer in everything that I do."

Phew. Well done. But you know what's coming next.

"What are your weaknesses?"

Bingo.

"I tend to tunnel vision. Sometimes missing nuances. And that's derived from me putting my head down to really get into the work and focus."

Her shoulders relaxed! She liked that response. Keep it up!

I studied her face as she read me, wondering if her skin was smooth due to her tight blonde bun, or if she did Botox. Izzy continued to ask me basic behavioral questions before digging into the core purpose of what brought me to the interview.

"I can tell that you've got a lot of energy, and I can also see that you're not afraid to get after what you want. But you've spent the last three years hopping around job to job. What makes you want a desk job?"

Hmmm…

"I want to excel at everything I do. First it was swimming. Then travel. But now I'm at a place in my life where I want security. I want to make real money. Structure my lifestyle. I'm ready to settle down and succeed in a position in sales."

Izzy scribbled every one of my words onto my resume, dousing it in red ink.

"Very well." Izzy put down her pen and stared up at me with her ice blue eyes.

"It looks like you've done a good job of living independently and figuring yourself out." She scooted her seat back, sliding it up against the wall behind her. "But I think you're still figuring it out."

Izzy stood up, shook my hand, and led me back to the lobby.

"We'll give you a call." Izzy waved me goodbye, and my heart dropped. I thanked the receptionist and stumbled back to my mom's car, dumbfounded.

What did any of that even mean? Of course, I'm still figuring it out! I just turned twenty-five! Half of that office just received their diplomas! I've traveled across the world, dammit. What makes her think I can't make a few phone calls?

Before I got too heated, I felt a buzz in my pocket. It was from the internal recruiter at the agency, inviting me in for one last interview. A half-day shadow and two oral evaluations. Oh, and scheduled for 8am the next morning.

Tomorrow? Like, in 16 hours, tomorrow? Crap, I've got 16 hours to get my shift covered or else I'm left with no job.

I called every server at the restaurant, begging someone to cover my lunch shift that next day, with no luck. The schedule hired extra staff to accommodate prospective crowds from an event next door, so I hoped my absence wouldn't be a big deal. I left messages for my restaurant manager to let her know that this corporate interview would be my last, and to apologize in advance for coming in late to work.

Hitting the gym first thing the next morning, I wrung out any excess nerves and slowly prepared for the big day. But just as I hopped out of the shower, I felt an uneasy, unsettling churn in my stomach.

The protein smoothie didn't help, the coffee certainly didn't help, and no number of Tums would stop the rumbling in my tummy. While I was not in dire pain, I did have diarrhea. Every visit to the bathroom forced me to face the mirror and affirm one thing:

Benefits and Healthcare.

In the office, I shook hands with dozens of smiling faces, all donning slacks and button-ups. When I made one last bathroom stop before the big interview, I noticed the sweat stains under my armpits reached towards my ribcage.

Fack! Not cool, Jen. Not cool. Why is everything *coming out today??*

The meeting ended like the other four, with empty grins, curt handshakes, and one last, "We'll give you a call."

When I returned to the car and reached for my phone, I received a late response from my restaurant manager.

Hey girl! I know you texted me about not being here for your shift, and I totally understand that you had your interview today. I hate doing this via text, but I have decided it would be the best for both of us if you no longer worked here.

I froze in the driver's seat and started to cry, recognizing my disposability.

When I got home, I smoked a bowl and stared at my ceiling for an hour until my mom returned home from work. With my eyes puffy from both the pot and my pity-party, I wasn't ready to tell her I got fired, but I didn't really have a choice. She sighed from the news and shrugged, "That's life and your responsibility. You got to get a job, Jenny."

Unemployed, my drive to create videos or start my memoir diminished under such scarce circumstances. Sure, I was under the care of my parents, but I had bills and a drug addiction. And while I lived rent-free, I paid the price of my parent's projections. "You're 25 and living with your parents! Don't you think that's weird?" They'd nag. "Don't you want a *real job* and a place of your own?" These comments often triggered a binge and purge, though living with them did make it harder to binge and purge without them noticing, which in a way, helped.

I was now purging one, maybe two times a week, mostly on the weekends while hungover or after a disappointing shift at the restaurant, where rude tables and small tips justified a feeding frenzy of shakes and waffle fries.

Five business days after my restaurant "lay off," I received an offer from the staffing agency. *Thank you, God.* I would trade an apron for a power suit, swapping weekend doubles on my feet to sitting behind a desk from 9-5, Monday through Friday. Or at least, that's what I thought.

In the same day my parents left to snow bird for the winter, I returned to the corporate office for the sixth time after those five interviews. *Everyone* shook my hand and offered a free lunch. That first week was fabulous as I shadowed coworkers, listened to training modules, and braked by noon. The open floor office contained rows of desks where chairs and computers lined side by side, separated by short barriers. We could easily see over the dividers as much as we could hear our coworker talk on the phone, all intentionally designed to readily give feedback or congratulate a coworker after a call.

"You ready to hop on the phone?" Mark, my manager asked on my first Friday. He was the quintessential suburban dad: loved to golf, gushed over his wife and toddlers, and low-key bragged about getting drunk on the weekends with his old frat buddies.

"I guess that's what I signed up for, huh?" I smiled nervously.

"I know it seems intimidating, but it's just like ripping off a band-aid. By Monday, you'll be blazing through your call sheets."

With Mark standing over my shoulder, I started dialing a number he gave me.

"Nothing's happening!" I panicked.

"You have to dial out with star 1…" Mark sighed with an eye roll.

The call went to voicemail, and I left a high-pitched message based on the script I received in my modules.

"Well, it's five on a Friday. Looks like you'll just have to make up for it with more calls next week." Mark teased.

Throughout those first two months, I dialed out fifty times a day, with a goal to have at least five constructive calls with people that qualified as leads. As a staffing agency, we were in the business of placing people into jobs that needed to be filled and filled fast. But time seemed to pass faster than my fingers could dial, and I ended up staying until 6:30pm most nights, which was common amongst the office. I came in early, following protocol yet hardly gaining traction with my leads. I was doing all the things they told me to do, but my needle moved me nowhere. I was hitting my outreach goals, but few of the people I headhunted converted into a placement, which was all that mattered to the business.

By December, my fingers and soul went numb. My coworkers were fine, my boss was fine. Mark was supportive and hadn't leaned over my shoulder since that initial phone call but got on my case a few times for looking "too casual" at work. This irked me, as some mornings I had hit snooze to recover from a previous night's binge and avoided the mirror all together. If my selection of flowy dresses were all dirty, leggings were the only pants that fit, but to my dismay, they didn't fly.

One outfit Mark commented on was from J. Crew and imitated what Izzy and other female managers wore. These comments always came on days I didn't have any face-to-face interactions, so what difference did it make on what I wore? And what's wrong with chambray?

I told myself it was time to go back to my personal projects. Realign my goals. Continue to heal my body and my eating disorder. While the severity and frequency of my purges vastly improved from Korea, I still felt a spiritual void. After an ugly purging relapse one weekend, I went to a Monday night OA meeting in Kansas. Unlike Korea, this church basement filled up with 30 English speaking people of all ages, of all body sizes, and in all stages of their healing. I loved being able to speak during my turn, as speaking up honestly to others who understood what I was going through was a new kind of purge. I wasn't so ashamed to speak this time. But the moment I got a sponsor, healing felt like a chore. The phone calls. The meetings. The Big Book readings and working the steps was too much to manage all at once, and soon enough I'd find myself driving through a custard stand for hot molten chocolate glazed over vanilla cream after having eaten two meals at home.

While I wasn't a regular, the meetings helped me to deepen my belief in a higher power. Each time I sat among other overeaters, I was reminded that I wasn't a bad person for all of the ugly things I did with food. However, I had a spiritual malady and a plagued ego. The long timers with decades of abstinence always spoke about ego. If I didn't keep it in check, I was a five-minute drive away from five candy bars I could buy for five dollars.

While I had come a long way from the years I felt out of control, I still drank and used and acted like an addict. The 9-5 I entered was really an 8-6, leaving me drained by the time I got to the gym, when I forced myself to run before smoking weed, eating dinner, and starting all over again the next morning. My weight had slimmed down about 20 pounds since moving home, putting me at a size 6. My work schedule helped me stick to a routine and meal plan for lunch, but any stressful day could send me back to a binge. The office culture split between ex-athletes still active as ever, and overweight colleagues eating fast food, pounding Red Bulls, and bringing doughnuts for everyone on 'Casual Friday's.' On those days, I'd cave with one, two, maybe three doughnuts if there were leftovers by noon. The office aura shifted on Friday's. Be it from the doughnuts or the denim or the fact that we were all working for the weekends. A drunken Friday night led to a three-day hangover, where I rot in bed beside empty food cartons. I worked hard in an industry I didn't understand, and played harder with girls who drank like I could. On this spectrum of extremes, I found no space to center, ground down and follow my dreams.

One Monday afternoon, I stopped by Bentley's to catch up. She had recently taken the plunge of quitting her job at a non-profit to pursue a full-time career as a yoga teacher. Bentley inspired me to dive back into my own yogic path, which I had practiced on and off since sixteen. As I took Bentley's classes, I learned how visceral yoga is and how much it impacts all facets of our lives. I admired Bentley for jumping all-in as a yoga teacher and yearned to work towards something I loved.

"How's work?" She asked.

Without letting me respond she added, "You hate it."

I stared at her, perplexed. I didn't like the word "hate," and I didn't want to mentally place myself in a position where I was miserable at work. Because during those first few months, I kept my head down every day to hit my quota. I was too focused on doing a good job, that I never assessed how much I actually liked said job.

"It's not what I expected. But I'm not sure what I was expecting, though. I just figured if your sister could do it and a handful of other kids from our high school could do it, then why can't I do it, too?" I sighed.

"Jenny, Reagan has been there for three years. She's still working her ass off and feels pressured even though she's climbed so high in the company. She is great at sales and I'm not saying you're not, but I also know how great of a writer you are, and how much you want to write your book." Bentley stared at me pensively as she defended her sister, took a beat, and continued.

"I wouldn't say this to anyone, because not everyone has it in them... I'm telling you, if you quit tomorrow, I know you'd be able to pick up gigs and hustle your butt off to write. You've got the drive to make it happen." Bentley said.

I stared out the window and sighed. "Yea... yea you're right, but I'm not ready. I just started there, and I can't quit so soon."

Bentley shot me a soft smile that said, "but you can, and one day, you will."

While Bentley and I talked about everything trauma and healing, yoga, and philosophy, pursuing our dreams and being fabulous while doing so, the conversations with my drinking buddies concerned bashing exes and procuring new boys. One Friday night, the gals and I gathered around a dinner table with bottles of flavored vodka placed in the middle and shot glasses scattered around the perimeter. Our host was describing the four dates she'd been on during the week as if taking a prescription for love.

"Jesus, how do you score so many dudes?" I asked, dumbfounded, and dying to know.

"I'm on Bumble for two weeks on, and two weeks off. That way, the pool refreshes and I'm not cycling through the same guys, resetting the algorithm." She said defensively and took a shot.

That night, my friends insisted I download the apps, then swiped generously for me as we drank through downtown Kansas City. Reluctantly, I "put myself out there," and really, *really* put out. Every date went smoothly, as it was easy to entertain myself with strangers. When the bar tab arrived, the man I had no interest in seeing again would pay, invite me back to his place, and take off both our clothes. There was never a second date. I did not want a second date. I just wanted to feel desired.

As the holidays came creeping, I decided dating apps weren't filling my cup and maybe men weren't supposed to be on my radar. New Year's was nearing, and I was ready for resolution.

I pledged to myself that 2018 Jenny would be different. 2018 Jenny would finish her book, she would cut the bullshit. No more drinking, no more drugs. No more dating retired frat boys on Bumble and *certainly* no more binging and purging.

No, 2018 Jenny wasn't going to mess around no 'mo. It was time to work hard and *focus.*

...

On Christmas Eve Eve, that being December 23rd, 2017, I ordered a pricey 40-minute cab into the city to bar hop with high school friends who were in town for the holidays. We caught everyone's lives up to speed by drinking feverishly, ordering sangria and champagne, IPA's and hard liquor. By midnight, we stumbled into the kind of dive bar that scares hipsters away when the scene gets too mainstream. There, my friend Mila visiting from Seattle pointed at a tall man in black leather, puffing on something sleek.

"Go ask if that's a weed pen." Mila nudged my elbow just as I lunged forward to complete her request.

"Hey" I smiled up at the cute guy with the vape, who's sleepy blue eyes were staring down at my chest.

"Yo" he smiled back, quickly flashing two rows of perfectly aligned, white teeth.

"Is that weed?" I nodded at his lips.

"Yea… here have a hit" He stared at my mouth as I took a large inhale, allowing something minty and sweet to fill my lungs.

Too drunk to know the difference, I later learned that I was hitting a Juul, which is a highly potent, electronic cigarette, and sadly not weed.

Ignoring this fib, I continued talking with this man, smoking with this man, and eventually sucking face with this man until a friend suggested we just go home.

Great idea.

Our limbs tangled in his bed. I desperately needed to pee and possibly vomit, but he had me pinned. While the pain in my temples sunk through my skull, something about his touch felt warm. It felt safe. As he opened his eyes, he greeted me with a kiss, held me tighter and went back to sleep.

Another hour passed as I assessed his thick brown hair pressed up against my armpit, with his head nestled on my boob. Surely, he couldn't be much older than a recent graduate given all the collegiate paraphernalia hanging in his small apartment. The unnamed boy finally got out of bed, bringing me water, coffee, and a bong to hit. The rush of weed turned me catatonic, and I realized I was extending my stay.

"I ought to go." I took out my phone to order a cab.

"Let me give you a ride home," He protested. "But before you leave, I've got something for you." His grin spread across his face as he turned around to dig in his closet. *Please don't lend me some dirty college tee shirt.* Instead, he pulled out a guitar.

> Strumming a familiar tune, he started singing:
> Hey, where did we go?
> Days when the rain came
> Down in the hollow
> Playin' a new game

He continued through the chorus of Van Morisson's "Brown Eyed Girl," kissed me, and grabbed the keys to his black Mustang. On the way to the suburbs, he stopped for a drink at a drive through, buying me a Powerade and reiterating "how much fun" he had had last night. I'm not one to get numbers after a one-night-stand, and figured this was our final goodbye. But just as I closed the car door, he rolled down his window and smiled, "Merry Christmas Jenny. Snap you later."

Jesus. Snapchat. Why are so many millennials still using this app? And as their primary mode of communication?

I rushed into my room before my parents could smell me and opened the app.

One Friend Added You!

Travis D.

Ah, that's right. His name was Travis. Thank you, Snapchat. Thank you.

Slipping out of my jumpsuit, I looked up at the mirror in dismay. My breasts were blue with bruises. Acute, dark marks spread across my chest. Turning my back in horror, I stopped to see - could that be – was that a bite mark? Did that dude *bite me?* First, he lies about his e-cig, then he bites me?

You're too high and too hungover for this. Take a nap, eat some food. You're on your last leg of this type of behavior, Jen. Because 2018 is the year you write your memoir. 2018 is right around the corner and baby, this year's for you.

The next weekend, it happened again. Drinking with my high school friends led to drunk Snapping, which led to "bumping into" Travis, which led to another sleepover. Travis was now a one-night-stand I had slept with twice, and it was time for me to go. Never once did I say, "see you later," "text me," or "until next time." Tomorrow was New Year's Eve, ringing in 2018. I had no time for boys, no need to fuck. Besides, if I was fooling around with a fuckboy, what did that make me?

Before I lifted my laptop to write, Travis came sliding into my DMs to ask me out on a date. Like a real date. Out in public during the day, unlike our past two encounters of meeting while intoxicated at 2am. Travis suggested we work out together at the mega gym I belonged to, using one of my monthly guest passes. Figuring this behavior was in alignment with my 2018 goals, I reasoned it was not weird at all to meet sober for the first time at a gym. After exercising, we hit his weed pen - a real one this time – and ate brunch, where he treated me to vegan pancakes. He was just as funny in the daylight as he was when we were drunk. However, we were high, so who's to say what was funny and what was fallacy. He then dropped me off at my parents' home and kissed me goodbye. No sex, no booze. Just an easy Saturday trip to the gym and a comfort meal. Like a real date, you know, like couples do. Having a man want to spend time with me was such a foreign feeling, that I let my infatuation override my writing. With Travis, I soon learned, my goals were mere scribbles lost in a journal.

Never having been outside the country himself, Travis was in awe of my travels. This baffled me considering he was financially stable to save up for a trip, though I understood that he had spent his adult life in nursing school. But Travis had ambitions to travel nurse starting that summer, in which I sincerely supported.

"You should go for it, Travis. Move as far away as possible. Just for a bit. It is so important for us to live outside our hometown, even if we come right back. You get a new perspective on things." I told him one Sunday morning.

"Yea, but babe... that'd mean missing you." He cooed. I blushed, but didn't let his words sink in. I liked the idea of dating Travis with a deadline, as Travis wasn't someone I could see myself marry, but surely enjoyed his company, his drugs, and his bed.

By February, Travis and I were seeing each other three nights a week, smoking, sipping, and having ample amounts of sex. My book remained untouched.

My 2018 goals of writing and sobriety evaporated in the whirlwind of dating a self-proclaimed addict. When I told him of my dad's early days of drinking and that I too had very addictive behaviors, Travis would stop the conversation to kiss me.

"It's comforting being with you. Another addict. Isn't it funny how we always find each other?" Travis said before hitting a weed pen one night in bed.

Something about this didn't sound right, but I nodded anyway. While I didn't want to fall victim to junkie love, I didn't want to go back to being alone, either. We continued seeing each other into the depths of winter, where the two of us played daringly through a series of snowstorms.

I blew more cocaine with Travis than the rest of my life in lines combined. By mid-January, we snorted the white every weekend and the occasional weeknights. I was under the spell of his drugs and the high of his affection. I soon found out that Travis took other drugs of his own: Adderall to keep him focused in the day, and at times, Viagra to keep him up at night.

One night, after plenty of blow and even more foreplay, Travis took an hour to get hard, and eventually came. He wrapped his arms tightly around my naked body, burying his head between my breasts. Lifting his lips to meet mine, he gasped.

"Wow, Jenny. I never get hard after Adderall, but I did tonight. Take that as a major compliment." He said. Not sure of what to say, I just smiled. Sure, it was flattering that I could turn him on without the help of Viagra, but I was tired of hearing how much he depended on drugs... for everything.

When he was sober, or at least I had hoped, Travis would Facetime me during our lunch breaks and texted me every morning, wishing me a beautiful day. I loved the undivided attention he gave me when we were together, but I hated it when he talked about his exes, when he took me to his coke dealer unannounced, or when he bailed at the last minute on dinner plans.

On the flip side, Travis became my accountability partner for my binging and purging, as I thought twice before digging into the pantry because I knew I'd be naked next to him soon. He praised and held and kissed my body, reminding me of its beauty, strength, and resilience. I adopted the care he showed me, slowly applying that care to myself.

One winter weeknight, he came over for our habitual date of drinking red wine and watching Netflix. Travis surprised me with Thai food, and I surprised him by saying he would have to dine alone, that I had already eaten.

"But babe, I got us spring rolls! Come on, have a little." He pleaded.

"Travis. It is so, so sweet of you to bring food, but I already ate and I'm not hungry. And I don't want to eat again because I'm trying to do a better job of listening to my body's hunger cues." I knew I was losing Travis with this vague response, and something told me it was time to tell him. We stood facing each other in my kitchen against the marble top island. I reached for his hands and investigated his wide, blue eyes.

"Travis. I want you to know something about me. Because I like you, I trust you, and I want you to understand me better."

I took a deep breath. I had been wanting to admit this to Travis since our first date over pancakes, but was afraid I'd come off as too much, too soon.

"Since I was eighteen, I've gone through a series of eating disorders. First, I was very anorexic, then I was bulimic. Today, I still struggle with restriction and binging, so I am careful about when I eat, and how much I eat. That's why I really like knowing in advance if you want to have dinner together, as having structure around eating helps with my recovery."

Travis smiled at me with patience, leaving space for silence. Before he spoke, Travis held me close and kissed my forehead.

"Thank you." He said.

"Thank you for sharing that with me Jenny. I can't imagine what you've gone through, and I know as a nurse how difficult it is to have an eating disorder. So again, thank you. Thank you for telling me." Travis leaned in to kiss me once more, igniting a spark between our lips. It was then I knew something about this confession changed our dynamic entirely.

Hours later as we nestled our bodies into the couch, Travis turned his head to kiss me once more while we watched American Horror Story. I looked into his cool eyes, which were floating above mine.

"I love you, Jenny," Travis professed. I was honored, but unsure of how to respond. I felt connected to Travis, but in love? That, I couldn't immediately decide, being pinned beneath him while a little drunk and high.

"You don't have to say anything, Jenny. Just know that I love you." He kissed me once more before turning towards the TV.

He loves me. Somebody loves me.

I was flattered. I felt seen. But I couldn't say it back right away; I was processing.

Later that night, he said it again during sex. Only this time, he asked me to say it back. Amid our lovemaking, I grabbed the back of his neck and dragged his face close to mine.

"I love you, too."

...

It was April, and I was in love. Or perhaps, infatuation. Travis kept me warm throughout the long winter we experienced in Kansas City, and I lusted over his heat. He had a way of speaking to me like I was the last woman on earth; the only person who seemed to matter. On the first sunny day of spring, my office celebrated a good quarterly performance with a half day of work, which happened to be Travis's day off. We got together and got drunk by 2pm. Around 3, he convinced me to pick up the remaining bag of molly I had bought the week prior.

"Molly? On a Thursday?" I asked with concern.

"Yea baby. I've never taken molly, and I'd only want to do it with you." Travis cupped his hands around my face.

"I love you," he said as kissed me.

We picked up the molly from my place, dividing what was left of my stash after an epic Lorde concert.

"It's not much. But we should still get a buzz." I told Travis as I broke a capsule into our palms.

For the rest of the day, Travis and I waltzed around town, playing frisbee golf and eating pizza. My subtle molly high made me feel so free, and I associated that freedom with Travis. Despite the drugs, he held me differently that night. He held me like Evan used to, like he didn't want to let go. I had missed this intensity. I didn't want to let go of it, either.

That next Friday morning at work, I was lucky to not be the only hungover employee. As I plodded through my tasks, I recounted the conversations between me and Travis, replaying yesterday's scenes, not letting a little headache dampen my spirits.

Then, unexpectedly, someone from high school messaged me about catching up. She was a mutual Facebook friend of Travis's, and I knew they had graduated from the same nursing school. I agreed and asked if she knew Travis, as he was "kind of my boyfriend." She said she did. She said that Travis wasn't her biggest fan, but she was happy for me.

Her text wasn't the response I was looking for, but I let it pass the second Travis texted me.

TRAVIS: Hey babe.

JENNY: Hey you. Sarah Miller just texted me and I told her you're my boyfriend, which makes you my boyfriend. Hope that's cool 😳 😶

Once I hit send, I realized that Travis and I had never talked about our dating status. The way I saw it, we had been seeing each other for four months, exchanging "I love you's" and texting every day. So yea, that made him my boyfriend. Besides, Travis always talked about his previous girlfriends, so why wouldn't I make the list?

He sent me back an upside-down smiling emoji, before sending this:

TRAVIS: Hey yea Sarah Miller is not my biggest fan, and I don't know how I feel about labels right now. After everything that happened with my ex and with me moving to travel nurse this summer, I just don't know if I'm emotionally available for a relationship right now.

I scooted my chair away from my desk, staring blankly at the white screen. My phone weighed heavier and heavier in my hand, until it slipped through my fingers. Instead of picking it up, I pushed myself out of my chair and headed to a bathroom stall so no one would see me panic.

Emotionally available?? You don't know if you're emotionally available? You can say that you love me, you can fuck me, and you can introduce me to your friends but when I ask to call you my boyfriend, you tell me you don't know if you're emotionally available. What does "I love you" even mean anymore?

I panted behind the stall, coming to terms with the situationship I had euphemized in my head. I had spent six years single as a choice, traveling the world, relishing my untethered life. 2018 was supposed to be a dedication of self-love, a time to clean up my act and write my book. Instead, I had handed my heart over to someone I never really knew--or at least never knew sober. All the fun came to a harsh stop once I realized I was being played.

Instead of responding to Travis's text, I cut him off on all my social media accounts. Reciprocating "I love you" caused enough emotional bruising, and I wouldn't let Travis cut any deeper.

"Don't you think you're being a little extreme?" He texted me after I told him I could not see him anymore. But every couple of weeks, he would weasel his way back through a sweet message, a phone call, and in late May, a visit to my new place. I had moved into a house with a childhood friend who gave me a fair rent in a nice neighborhood. My parents were pleased that I had moved out and into this small, three-bedroom home with a big backyard and two of my roommate's rowdy dogs. However, my roommate wasn't home when Travis's Mustang pulled up in the driveway.

"Wow, Jen. You live so close." He said as he kissed me in the doorway.

Yea, dude. I was always planning to move in the Spring, and we were supposed to stay together until your nursing contract started in mid-June. Remember that plan? Or were you too drunk to pay attention every time we talked?

That evening, I got a bit of the closure I was looking for. He apologized for the discrepancy over our relationship status and attested his adoration for me with kisses. Lots of kisses. He took my shirt off to feel me up and I started reaching for his zipper.

"Oh, Jen. I can't have sex. I'll get too attached."

I backed off, stunned. *Too attached? Do you remember how we met?*

A moment later, he rolled over to pin me down, kissed my neck and dove down to bite my stomach.

"Woah! What the hell?" I yelled.

I stared down at the teeth marks near my belly button. He looked at me with eyes that wouldn't say sorry. I grabbed my top and escorted us to the front door for one more goodbye.

I hated that he bit me, trying to leave his mark. I hated how much I loved him being there, in my bed and in my arms. All the while, I knew how twisted it was, to long for a taste of someone who would not commit, and instead allow him to leave with a taste of me.

Three weeks passed without hearing from Travis. This lightened up my mental load to revel in the summer. Boys -and unfortunately, writing - were the last things on my mind during reunion trips to see Ava in Toronto and Brooklyn at Bonnaroo. It was now late June and the beginning of my birthday week, when I received an unknown text from a number I had deleted weeks ago.

UNKNOWN: It's my last week in KC. Wanna hang?

I knew it was foolish to comply, but so was falling for someone I had never known in a sober state. Alas, I told Travis I would come over at six, until six came around and Travis had something better in mind.

Jenny: I'm heading over.

Travis: Nah I changed my mind.

What. The. Fuck.

Jenny: You're a shithead.

Travis: Real classy, Jen.

Jenny: Travis, breaking plans with me is hurtful. It hurt when you did that to me in the winter and it hurts now. You're leading me on and stealing away my time and it's a shitty way to remember you.

My phone started ringing.

"Jenny." He was drunk.

"Jenny. I need you to know. That I love you. I think you are the perfect girl, Jenny. But..."

But?

"But I'm not sexually attracted to you. And Jenny..."

And what??

"I have a girlfriend."

The conversation went silent. Everything went numb. My tongue swelled up and my heart began to sting.

"Jenny. This girl... I was never that attracted to her at first but now..."

Wait, are you trying to explain why you like your girlfriend to break up with me... again?

"Travis, you were over just weeks ago, kissing me in my bed. And now you have a *girlfriend?* Don't bother going into detail, please. But tell me if you were with her when you were with me."

'When you were with me.' That last line left a bitter taste in my mouth, as I questioned what our existence as a couple even meant to Travis.

"No, Jenny. Of course not. I loved you. I still love you. I'm just not sexually attracted to you."

You already said that part.

"Besides, it doesn't really matter because I'm moving, and I don't know if my girlfriend and I will even stay together."

Ok, Travis. You're moving to Warrensburg, Missouri. A town where the fun thing "to-do" is visiting to Kansas City. You could commute if you really wanted to, but you're right, it doesn't really matter.

"Jenny. You're the perfect girl. And I love you. But we can't be together... Because I have a girlfriend."

Why was he wasting his breath to end things with me, *again*? He could have inhaled a dozen Juul hits over the course of this redundancy. Our fling ended the moment he admitted he was "emotionally unavailable." Once he disclosed that message in April, he shot a dagger into my chest. And as I listened to his words on this call, that dagger turned. In hindsight, this was a blessing and the sting helped me wake up from his toxic fumes. This relationship was over, and the dagger was removed, but I would need some time to heal the wound.

The next day at work, my director Izzy took one look at my face and led me into her office.

"What's going on?" She asked.

I took a deep inhale and unleashed the flow of ugly cries that were streaming since Travis's phone call.

"The guy I've been seeing...*sniff*... broke up with me last night... *sniff*... said he wasn't attracted to me... *sniff*... and said he has a new girlfriend!" My crying was gross, excessive, and amusingly unprofessional. So be it! I was distraught beyond measure. My serious, sales-driven boss dropped her shop talk and got real.

"Jenny. Let me tell you something. I once dated a man for five years and when he broke up with me, he also said he wasn't attracted to me. Which wasn't true, it was just an excuse. But you know what? That break up got me in the best shape of my life and I met my husband shortly after. I'm sorry you are going through this, and I don't want you to have to go through it at work. Please take a personal day. See you tomorrow."

I looked up at Izzy through my tears, mumbled "thank you" and slumped home, continuing to cry in my bedroom. Curling up in a fetal position on my bed, I made sure to let out every belch before my roommate returned home from work.

I couldn't understand why I was in so much pain, as Travis and I were over months ago. I hated how he played me, but what I hated the most was that I saw this coming after our first night together. Travis waved every red flag, *bleeding* bad boy behavior. But once I asked myself to make 2018 a year for writing and refraining from my vices, I drifted towards Travis's warning lights like a moth. Instead of working on myself and my book, I participated in this dumpster fire of a relationship, but only I got burned.

Between the crying spells, I prayed and prayed to not turn to food. When my hands weren't in prayer, I picked up my pen to journal so I wouldn't grab my car keys for a binge. I took initiative on that personal day by setting an appointment with a referred therapist, walking my roommate's dogs, and of course, smoking a lot of weed. With an hour to kill before my roommate returned home, something spoke to me as I waited for her company.

Write it out.

I opened a Google Doc on my iPad and started typing. When I finally looked back up at the screen, I smiled for the first time all day:

Confused

I am not blind
But I cannot see
Why you spend your time
Wasting away with me
You said I was your best friend
And that is a lie
I believed you could make me happy
And so I let you try
You didn't make me happy
I learned
I make myself happy
But having you still helped
As you showed me the love
I was hiding from myself
You let me wear your smile.

During this grieving period, I wrote poems every day. I typed on my phone from under my desk, and behind the wheel at stop lights just to get a thought out. After work, poems poured out of me. I was writing for myself, and I was writing to Travis, with the impression that what I had written would never be read. That was up until I was told that what I was writing wasn't half bad.

"Jenny! You need to put this shit on Instagram!" Bentley and I were on her couch when I read my poems aloud for the first time. She grabbed my wrist and placed her other hand on her heart while I shared my poems:

Lazy
With you,
Every Sunday was lazy
I could lay around for hours
Effortlessly loving you

Life of the Party
You were a glass half full kind of guy
After all
It was never empty

Stimulants
We drank and we laughed
And blew more lines
We went to the casino
And I blew on your dice
When we got home
I tried to blow you
But your dick doesn't work
Not like it's supposed to
What keeps you awake won't get you up

"Seriously, Jen. That's how Rupi Kaur made it. She kept posting her poems on Instagram and now she tours the world."

I laughed off Bentley's response initially, but back home, I gave her suggestion some careful consideration. My Instagram was evolving from cute one-liners and emojis to captions of more reflective, more meaningful messages. I was posting about my mental health, and followers appreciated my honesty. But to post poetry? Now *that* was simply too vulnerable.

During dinner with my high school friends, I zipped my legs together under my seat to avoid fidgeting, impatiently waiting for a chance to share my writing. Everyone at the table had already read and reverenced Rupi Kaur's *Milk and Honey,* so I was eager to ask their opinion about a piece:

"Guys! I've been writing away and I got a good one for you, are you ready?"

They all stared at me blankly.

"Ok…" I set the tone, silencing my audience in a small corner of the restaurant.

Empty

I don't miss your sex

I miss having you inside me

"Well… What do you think?" I asked my three friends, now staring into the ether.

"Yea… I mean it hits hard," one friend said, looking somber.

"I could never say that," said the second, shaking her head.

"Okay… but you're not the one saying it, I am!" I responded proudly. I kept on smiling, keeping my cheeks tight to avoid any hints that I was annoyed by the last response. I was hoping for a little bit more... receptivity. Like Bentley had shown me days ago.

"I won't post this one online, but I'm thinking about sharing some others on Instagram. It just feels good to write them, and I'm sure someone will relate…" I said, looking at my third friend, who was an avid reader and closet writer.

"Jenny, your poems are beautiful and I'm sure it's cathartic for you, but you don't have to post your poems on Instagram for them to be valid. You can always keep your writing to yourself." She said sitting erect, setting her fork on top of her salad as carefully as she had chosen her response.

I bit my tongue and tried changing the topic. Maybe these friends were not ready for my poetry. Maybe hearing something raw from someone they knew was different than reading a poem from the acclaimed Rupi Kaur. Or maybe I wasn't emotionally ready for their unfavorable responses as I sought out validation. Therefore, I sought out a professional.

For a hundred dollars a session, I saw a therapist after that last call with Travis, to talk about heartbreak and a bit about eating. She was kind, supportive and extremely helpful, but too expensive to see regularly. So, on our third and last appointment, I mentioned my writing.

"I've been writing poems every day. It's helping me detach from Travis and see our relationship in a different light, but writing about him makes me have to think about him, which is something I'm working hard not to do."

"Why don't you write about something else?" she suggested.

I pondered her comment, raising my brows to ask, *'now, what would that be?'*

"What else is bothering you, Jenny?" she probed.

I immediately blurted out, "I hate my job."

Woo! Did I just admit that aloud?

The therapist nodded, waiting for me to elaborate.

"My boss is on my ass for the dumbest shit. I've gotten in trouble a couple of times for my clothes - my J. Crew outfits! And so many of my projects fall through because of things outside my control."

Let it out, Jen. Let it out.

"Why don't you write about work, then?" she said just as our time was up.

Ah, yes. Why don't I write about work...

My first poem set the stage for the finale of my corporate career:

The artist inside me would rather starve
Than stare at the screen which feeds me

Every minute of every stale day in that office provided me with material, and every cell in my being begged to leave so I could let those words free. I tried disassociating. Masking up into corporate mode for ten hours a day, unveiling into an artist at night. I would wake up around 5am each morning, work out and prepare breakfast as I read poetry with my coffee. Preparing for a momentous day, this optimism vanished once I slipped my flats on and reached for the door. Each time I stared out at my newly financed, emerald green, Fiat 500, the coffee churned in my stomach. I did not want to get in my car. *And I loved that car.* But that car symbolized my commute. And that commute stripped me away from myself.

...

"Jenny, is there anything going on that we should know about?" Izzy asked me one Friday afternoon in September. She called me and Mark into her office for an impromptu meeting, where Mark and I sat on a bright red couch, facing her white, leather chair.

"Ah... No. I had some personal issues in the summer, but I'm better now. I know my numbers have dropped but I keep hitting my call goals... I've just been having a tough time converting them into placements..." I looked into Izzy's piercing eyes to tell her I was trying, then down at the floor to indicate it was only a matter of time before giving up.

Mark sat there in silence, awkward as Izzy interrogated.

"Jenny... there's something missing from you. I can't quite tell what it is, but I'm not seeing the drive from you like I did last fall. Is there something you need from me or Mark to help you with your placements?" Izzy clamped her hands together on the desk and leaned forward as she tilted her head, probing.

"I'm just... not feeling very creative here." I hesitated to continue, knowing I had sparked a concern the moment the "C" word left my lips.

"This is a creative job!" Izzy reflexed back as her cheeks blushed. "You must get creative in finding great candidates. Interviewing is *extremely* creative." Her pink, buttercream lips lined her wide, sharp smile. I tried staying coy. The position I thought I signed up for – one which challenged my communication and personable skills - had now become a grueling task of repetitive phone calls. Same shit, different days.

Sales is an artform, no denying that. But I didn't want to sell myself short of the gifts I'd been handed and neglect the creative energy I had cultivated since college. I stormed out of Izzy's office once she finished evaluating my plateauing performance and drank the weekend away.

The following Monday at work, I made fake phone calls and left ghost voicemails before 11am, when I slid out of the office for a long lunch break with a high school friend.

"Jenny, I am not telling you to quit your job. But you seem miserable." My girlfriend said as we ate acai bowls from an outdoor patio. The sun dried my tears that had been streaming since I left for lunch. I knew she was right. I had lost my spark a year ago, replacing ambition with toxic men, drinking, and drugs. Every morning when I would stare at my car, I stepped out of my true form to fit into the employee template. I tried to copy and paste the system, but something was wrong in my code. I started drinking on my lunch breaks, smoking weed on Fridays. I faked a funeral because I knew no one would believe me if I called in sick. Over Labor Day Weekend, I took a five day 'staycation' to write poetry and apply to new jobs. I didn't have any leads or a direction of where I wanted to go, but I knew I had writing material, and perhaps this meant I could return to my 2018 goal of finishing a book.

I had no backup plan. I had no savings. But I also had nothing left to offer to my staffing company, as a year of working behind a desk had sucked me dry. My friend was right: I was miserable. I returned to the office after lunch with the conviction to change. My stint in a pencil skirt was over. I hung my head low and limped into Mark's office.

"I can't do this anymore."

Mark took a big breath, then smiled. He was relieved he would no longer have to manage my unhappiness.

"Very well. It's been a pleasure working with you. I'm glad you've made the decision to find something that suits you." He paused, as if to contemplate his own resignation.

"I'll let Izzy and HR know, but just hang here for a bit. I'll bring you your sign-off papers, so you don't have to talk to anyone out there. Feel free to leave after you speak to Izzy. You can come back this evening to clean up your desk." Mark returned with a file for me to initial, gave me a hug and sent me to Izzy's office. There, she drilled a look between my eyes that could have split me in half - if I wasn't already broken.

"Thank you for everything, Izzy, I..."

"This job isn't for everyone. I'm sorry it took so long for us to see that this job wasn't for you. Good luck out there." Izzy lowered her stare back to her computer as I saw myself out of her office. I deflected glares as I tried to leave without drawing attention to my departure. But I was bombarded with side eyes as my ex-coworkers watched another quitter leave, then looked back at their laptops to fuel the machine.

Once I arrived home, I immediately opened my Google Doc and began typing.

Promises

They told me pencil skirts would write my success story

The next night, I enlisted friends to close the bars down with me on a Wednesday. By Friday, I took MDMA at a rave, kissed strangers and expressed to the crowd that I was a free agent. But when Monday came along, I woke up in a panic after burning through the first week of my two-week payout, and no amount of drugs or alcohol could mend my internal discord. I turned to writing to rid me of such malaise, only to be mocked by the blank page.

Each flash from the blinking cursor struck like a ticking time bomb. The free time I had longed for now trapped me in anxiety. How could I possibly write poems when I had rent to pay? Had I made a huge mistake?

I was forced to recalibrate. I dialed down the drinking and prioritized my health. I worked front desk at a gym in the morning, data entry at a start-up by the day, and promoted liquors at grocery stores on the weekends. I freelanced in editing and copy writing and dog sat for friends, family, and trusting strangers I met on the internet. Once again, I moved back in with my parents. They weren't thrilled, but at least they could monitor my partying. I inundated my ears with self-help audiobooks, listening to "Big Magic" on repeat while taking long walks in the woods. In "Big Magic," Elizabeth Gilbert discourages burdening our art by relying on it for money. We create because we must. If we happen to make money, then that's a lovely bow on top of the gifts we've been given. Whatever we do as artists, we should never, *ever* quit our day jobs for the sake of writing a book.

Welp.

That fall, I made self-care my full-time job, vehemently writing between part-time gigs. I meditated, I stretched. I affirmed nice things to myself in the mirror. And no matter what, I showed up to write. Somedays, all I could muster was editing an old line, but I was ready to catch inspiration when it arrived. I noticed that beyond boys and bosses, I had not addressed my relationship with my body. The one thing that will *always* stick with me. The thick skin that harbors my heart and soul.

My connection with my body revealed an ecosystem of topics I needed to dissect on paper. I was an anorexic, an orthorexic, a bulimic, an overeater, an over-exerciser, a woman with body dysmorphia and a human who had forgotten how to love themselves. This work cultivated a hunger within me. Not for food, but for justice in honoring the vessel I had treated with disdain.

In the final months of 2018, I solely focused on poems about "The Voice Inside My Head." Such prose depicted behaviors of picking apart my plate and isolating myself in shame. This initially grueling practice allowed me to look at my past without holding onto the pain. As I released through words what I had hoarded in emotions, I cried. I cried at home, at libraries and at cafes. I could hardly see the screen through my incessant blubbering. But I didn't care. I was taking care of myself by normalizing weeping in public across the Greater Kansas City area.

This emotional inventory assessed what I had done to myself, my body, and my loved ones when ignoring their needs while consumed by disease. I had to look at myself. Not in the mirror, but in my actions, motives, and resentments. I couldn't just compare my present day from old photos online, yet part of my process was reeling back the timeline. From a double zero to a double chin, I imagined hugging each version of myself within. Every era of Jenny experienced change and trauma, shortcomings, and growth. From thin Jenny to fat Jenny, I loved them both. I let go of the girl who ate carrot sticks for dinner and forgave the girl who let an extra ounce of broccoli spiral into a night of bulimia.

That girl who starved herself so she could fit into whatever mold society told her to be. The girl who people pleased. If I never grew out of that girl, I would still be a size 2 and counting every calorie. I would work in HR or realty and lock down a man to marry me. I would keep my social media alive with consistent posts of filtered photos, baiting for followers to comment, "I want your life" and #squadgoals.

But I grew out of that girl. I got hungry. I no longer cared for my appearance to be the only asset of my identity. I wanted something to offer to the world. Rather roam it aimlessly. So I practiced staying still, meditating. I listened to learn that we aren't everything we think. I watched the thoughts float by slowly.

I grew out of that girl.

But that girl is still a part of me.

...

"Oh... This one gets personal."

The emcee at the writers' conference had finally pulled my index card for the "Ask the Agent" panel. In a small auditorium at my local library, the emcee sneered down at my question, smirked, and continued:

"'Do you represent poets?' And in parenthesis it says, 'about purpose, love and eating disorders.'"

"I only represent *novelists* that write poetry, so if I haven't worked with you before, I won't be selling your poems" said the New York City agent, unamused.

The grin on my face wore off after hearing this response and I slumped into the main corridor after the breakout session. There, a bald, older gentleman stepped in front of me, catching my attention.

"You a writer?" he asked.

"Yes! I'm almost finished with my manuscript" I said, delighted by his interest.

"Science-fiction?" he asked.

"No, poetry," I smiled back.

"Well..." he snickered. "...Good luck."

He kept on laughing and walked away. I did my best not to chuck my backpack at him and instead, resisted tears as I headed for the bathroom.

How could he mock me like that! Ugh. I'll show him. The next time sees me will be from the back of the line for my book signing of "Emotionally Bankrupt!"

That weekend I wrote a couple more poems, my foreword, and my afterword. I wouldn't let some strange man ridicule my dreams, so I pushed through my personal publication deadline and hit *print*.

My poetry was raw, and it was me. It was the first time I felt proud enough to say, "I let society dictate my dreams: being skinny. I skipped meals and threw up - *a lot*. I have loved men who didn't love me back and you know what? That's ok."

And while "Emotionally Bankrupt" was not my memoir, writing and releasing my poetry affirmed myself as an author. I did something for myself and shared it with others. I did something for myself that took all my energy, but cost nothing.

When I self-published the book on April 1, 2019, on Amazon, I was ecstatic for weeks. I rented out rooms in coffee shops, bars, and bookstores for free or next to nothing, hosting readings for the public and private parties.

One local bookstore donated their upstairs venue space for a two-hour event, waiving the $60 fee because it was my first reading. My parents, my brother, my cousins, aunts, and uncles came, along with my grandma and grandpa who drove in from St. Louis.

Between the lines, I caught glimpses of my father's swollen eyes as I expressed my side of anorexia, and my mom's fair skin flood with red whenever I mentioned sex.

Hugs and photos concluded the reading, documenting an afternoon of love and support. Then my dad, who never asked much about my writing, pulled me aside from the crowd of other Martins. He started crying. Something I hadn't seen since his mom passed away when I was in high school and said something I hadn't heard since my college graduation.

"I'm proud of you, Jenny."

He diverted quickly to dab his wet eyes, gave me a hug, and returned to his seat to take a sip of his iced tea.

I had not healed my bulimia at this point. And while I don't throw up my meals anymore, I am still not healed. Because healing is not finite. We are never heal-*ed*. We are in recovery, and remission requires daily maintenance. Even if I abstain from binging and purging for the rest of my life, I will still be a bulimic. A recovering bulimic.

"Emotionally Bankrupt" was not a book I had always felt called to write. It was a response to a grim time in my life. And while writing poetry helped me to look at myself with honesty, it only brushed the surface of much deeper work. I would need to start my memoir, "Jenny Eats the World: Tales of a Traveling Bulimic" to truly see all the chaos I have caused and all the addictions I possess. I would need to get sober to thoroughly understand the consequences of my self-destruction. Spoiler alert: sugar and substances are not my problem. I am.

I published "Emotionally Bankrupt" during a yoga teacher training, which propelled profound behavioral changes with my purging, partying, and promiscuity. But we don't have time to touch on that now, so I'll leave you with this:

Staying silent about the things that make you feel crazy and ultimately make you go crazy will kill you. And if you try to escape your crazy, your crazy will come back and catch you. But you're not crazy. Not even a little. Rather, you're built up with energy that is dying to come out, and luckily, no one has to die when you do so.

You can write. You can pray. You can call someone you trust and please, try finding people who have gone through similar experiences as you when venting about the things that weigh you down. We've all been told to act and dress and live a certain way, when really, we need to listen to ourselves. But we get confused at times, when depression and anxiety try to talk louder than our own intuition. That's where writing comes in. Because writing helps us find our voice. To speak our truth, to ask for help.

Thank you for listening to my story. As writing it has helped me to shape my past in a way that no longer cripples me with shame, and reliving each chapter proves that I have survived each and every one of my darkest days. I hope by reading a bit about my path, you are inspired to go forth and draft up the life of your dreams. Of love, of travel, and of ever-evolving, perpetual healing.

ABOUT THE AUTHOR

Jennifer Martin is a New York based, Kansas City native with an affinity for all things foreign. While she has dabbled in many vocations, her first creative title was that of an escape artist. Having lived across three continents in her early twenties, she has now settled into America's melting pot as an author and performing artist, sharing her story of addiction and eating disorder recovery.

You can follow along in Jennifer's unfiltered, online life at:
@jennifermartin.live
www.jennifermartin.live

You may share this memoir via:
@jenny.eats.the.world

www.ingramcontent.com/pod-product-compliance
Lightning Source LLC
Chambersburg PA
CBHW050854150626
46549CB00013B/1619